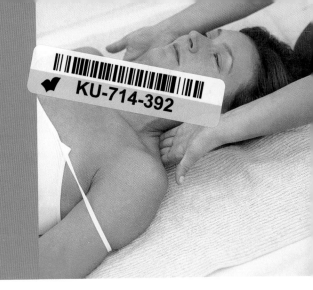

Massage
Basics

Wendy Kavanagh

hamlyn

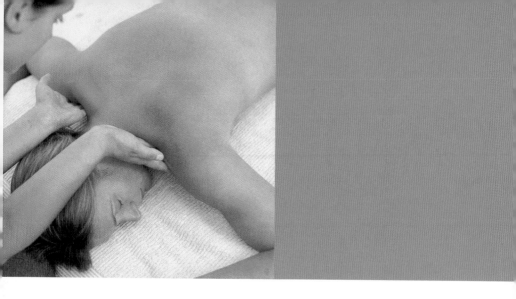

First published in Great Britain in 2004
by Hamlyn, a division of Octopus Publishing Group Ltd
2–4 Heron Quays, London E14 4JP

Copyright © Octopus Publishing Group Ltd 2004

Distributed in the United States and Canada by
Sterling Publishing Co., Inc.
387 Park Avenue South, New York, NY 10016–8810

ISBN-13: 978-0-600-61007-6
ISBN-10: 0-600-61007-1

A CIP catalogue record for this book is available from the
British Library

Printed and bound in Spain

10 9 8 7 6 5 4

This book is extracted from *Home Health Massage*,
published in 2002

It is advisable to check with your doctor
before embarking on any massage
programme. This book should not be
considered a replacement for
professional medical treatment; a
physician should be consulted in all
matters relating to health and particularly
in respect of pregnancy and any
symptoms which may require diagnosis
or medical attention. While the advice
and information in this book is believed
to be accurate and the step-by-step
instructions have been devised to avoid
strain, the publisher cannot accept legal
responsibility for any injury or illness
sustained while following the massages.

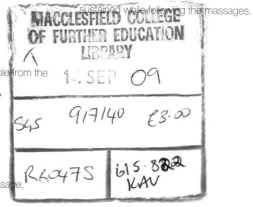

Contents

Introduction

One definition of touch is 'to make physical contact, to affect emotionally' and, interestingly, touch is the first sense we develop. By the sixth week of pregnancy the tactile sense has already started to evolve in the foetus, and this will create the basis for all our other tools of communication. As newborns we touch to survive, and the quality of the touch we receive as we grow up will determine our levels of self-esteem, our ability to form lasting relationships with others and our capacity to be comfortable with ourselves, both physically and mentally.

Touching for Health and Happiness

Massage has been practised for thousands of years and its effects have been well documented, telling us clearly that it is good for us – regular practice means we become calmer, healthier and happier. So how does it work?

Under the skin, massage causes complex processes to start: hormones and 'signal substances' transmit messages to the brain and back again, some stimulating and others calming. Touch is known to increase the level of oxytocin, the hormone that makes us relax, which in our fast-paced modern lives is a necessary means to restoring balance in our physical, emotional and spiritual well-being.

How did it all Begin?

Massage in some form is the earliest known therapeutic art, with an extensive and well-documented history. Before that we can only speculate that there was an equally strong instinct to stroke or touch the human body.

The earliest Chinese references to massage are in the medical text known as the *Nei Ching*, from the 25th century BC, and by the following

---

WHY MASSAGE?

- The word 'massage' comes from the Greek *massein*, 'to knead', which is descriptive of a technique that forms part of massage as it is practised today.
- 'Therapeutic touch' also comes from the Greek *therapeutikos*, relating to the effect of medical treatment.
- Until the 19th century, instead of 'massage' Americans used the term *frictio*, from the Latin meaning 'rubbing' or 'friction'.
- In India the art of massage was known as *shampooing*, in China as *cong-fou* and in Japan as *ambouk*.
- The term 'Swedish massage' is often used today, referring to the work of Per Henrik Ling, a native of Sweden who was a pioneer of the massage movement in the Western world (see opposite).

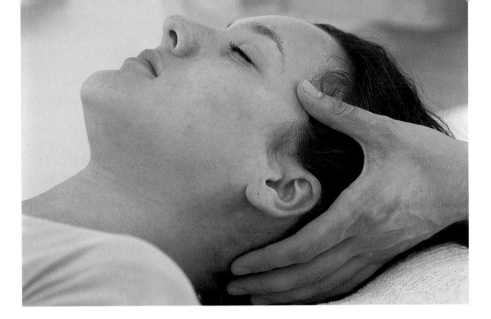

century the art appears to have spread across the civilized world because wall paintings depicting massage and reflexology have been found in a physician's tomb in Saqqara, and references by Egyptian, Persian and Japanese physicians to the benefits and usefulness of massage appear.

There are continued references to massage throughout history, from the books of the Indian *Ayur Veda* in the 19th century BC to Homer, as well as Greek medical texts of the 5th century BC. The Romans, too, had various uses for massage: gladiators were given regular treatments to ease muscle fatigue and pain, Julius Caesar was 'pinched' all over as a daily treatment for neuralgia, and the 1st century AD physican Tiberius believed it to be a cure for paralysis.

The use of massage continued in the Middle East and Far East, although it was suppressed in the West during the Middle Ages. The 10th-century Arab philosopher and physician Ali Abu Ibn Szinna extolled the health-promoting properties of massage combined with hydrotherapy, stating that it helps to disperse muscle by-products not expelled by exercise.

In the 16th century, massage began to make a strong comeback in the West and many prominent physicians incorporated it into their approach, including Amrose Pare, medical advisor to four French kings.

The best-known development in massage took place early in the 19th century. Per Henrik Ling, a Swedish gymnast, combined his knowledge of philosophy and gymnastics with massage techniques acquired during his travels to China. This combination of five basic strokes became known as the 'Swedish Movements' and is practised in much the same way today.

The discipline spread very quickly: the first college offering massage on the curriculum was established in 1813, and the first book in English on the Swedish Movements, written by Dr Mathias Roth, was published in 1850.

The biggest turnaround came in the 1960s and 1970s, with advocates considering massage to be a powerful means of promoting personal growth. This idea emanated from the Esalen Centre in California, where massage is used intuitively, connecting mind, body and spirit.

In the 21st century, massage has become a mainstream complementary therapy and also a part of integrated medicine as we know it. It is used throughout society on many levels and has a very important role to play in maintaining a healthy everyday life.

Preparation

Massage is easy to learn: let your instincts guide you and you will be able to sense where to touch, how to touch and for how long. There are just a few basic guidelines to follow to ensure a comfortable and beneficial treatment. During massage there is an interaction of touch and response, which means that the giver has to prepare to give while the receiver must allow them to do so. Only when these conditions are right can this two-way flow be effective.

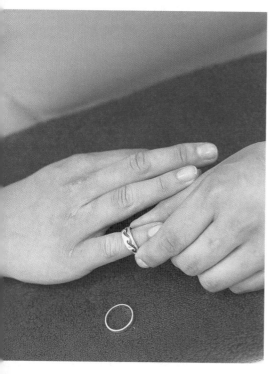

It is not a good idea to give a massage if you are stressed or tense or if you are not in full health, as your energy levels will be depleted. Both before and during the treatment, be aware of your breathing but do not try to change it.

Wear comfortable footwear and clothes. Choose something with short sleeves or roll them up out of the way. Take off any noisy jewellery, which can be very distracting, and remove your watch and any rings.

You cannot massage with long nails, and rough skin will feel very abrasive, so get out the nail clippers and hand cream. If you have long hair, tie it back to avoid it distracting either of you. Remember that you will be working very close to your partner, so if you have recently indulged in strong-flavoured food or drink use a mouthwash or breath freshener.

The Receiver

It is often much more difficult to receive massage than to give: the ability to trust and let go sometimes also has to be learned. Be receptive to the touch, allow the giver to move your limbs for you when required, and let them know if anything is uncomfortable or when a stroke is particularly effective.

Sometimes massage can release pent-up emotions. If this happens, there is nothing wrong – do not fight the feelings or become embarrassed, but simply let them go.

The Giver

You must choose actively to give your time to someone. If your mind is elsewhere, your partner will sense this and the massage will not be pleasurable for either of you. Care, sensitivity and respect are very important requirements, so your mind should be freed up to give your partner your full attention.

Before the massage begins, remember to take off all your jewellery, including earrings, and if you are wearing contact lenses you may prefer to remove them for comfort and safety, especially if the giver is going to work on your head or face.

With close friends and family, the receiver may be happy to undress to underpants; otherwise, only the areas of the body that are being worked on need be exposed at any one time. The ideal is to work free of clothing restrictions, but the massage environment is not always appropriate for this.

As with the giver, do not forget that fresh breath is a must, so use a mouthwash before receiving your massage.

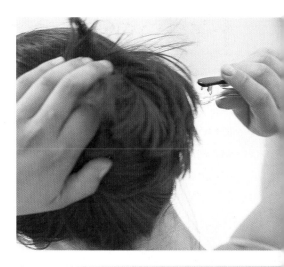

WHEN NOT TO MASSAGE

In general, massage is safe. Trained therapists are able to treat everyone from premature babies to the terminally ill, but if any of the following apply, you should not massage, or should take great care as directed below:

- Anyone weak or clinically exhausted – for example, suffering or recovering from a viral infection.
- Anyone who has a high temperature or is suffering from a contagious disease.
- Anyone who has infectious skin complaints, such as scabies, herpes and warts.
- Anyone who has a serious medical condition such as cancer, heart disorders or thrombosis.
- Do not massage the site of a recent fracture, strain or sprain. In these cases, work one joint above.
- Do not massage directly where there are skin surface problems, such as scar tissue,

bruising, tender or inflamed areas and varicose veins. You can, however, work with care above the site and, of course, on other unaffected parts of the body.
- Do not massage during the first trimester of pregnancy and thereafter avoid very deep pressure, particularly on the lower back and inside leg from ankle to groin.
- After surgery, wait for 12 months following major operations and six months following minor procedures. Scar tissue should then be fully healed, but if in doubt seek medical practitioner approval.

It is also not advisable to receive massage if you have recently eaten a heavy meal or have been drinking quantities of alcohol, as this will make the experience very uncomfortable and may produce unpleasant after-effects. The general rule is to trust your own judgement and common sense and, if in any doubt, check with a doctor.

Oils, Lotions and Potions

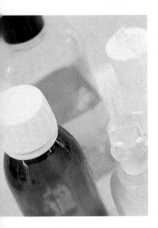

Most massage treatments require the use of a lubricant in order to allow your hands to work smoothly and evenly over the skin without breaking the rhythm. This usually takes the form of oil, although lotions, creams and sometimes talcum powder can be used if you prefer.

In general approximately 50ml (2½fl oz) is needed for a whole body massage. It may take a few tries to get it right: most people tend to use too much at first, which means you will not be able to make good contact. Your aim is to use just a thin film, which will be absorbed into the skin after the treatment.

Household Oils

You can use oils that you keep at home in the kitchen cupboard – sunflower, grapeseed and vegetable oils make excellent carrier or 'base' oils, as they are known professionally. If you want to pamper your partner, almond oil is a little costly but a real treat, particularly when used on the face. There is no need for you to worry about nut allergies because you are only applying oil externally and the penetration is superficial. However, some baby oils that include lanolin may cause an adverse skin reaction and tend to be absorbed less easily.

Essential Oils

These oils are very concentrated and powerful; many have contraindications, and unless you are a trained aromatherapist stick to the 'safe' oils, such as lavender and chamomile, especially for pregnant women.

Never apply essential oils neat to the skin, but always mix with a carrier oil in the ratio of 1 drop essential oil to 2ml (scant ½ teaspoon) carrier oil. For example, 10ml (2 teaspoons) sunflower oil would allow you to use a maximum of 5 drops of essential oil. Mix only enough for the treatment, as oils exposed to the atmosphere oxidize and become rancid.

Store aromatherapy oils in dark bottles so as not to destroy their properties. Always read the instruction leaflet carefully, and if in doubt consult a trained aromatherapist or use plain oil.

There are now so many pre-blended oils available, covering all types of occasions and moods, that purchasing one of these is often the safest and most economical way of enhancing your massage treatment.

Lotions, Creams and Powders

Massage lotions and creams are also available, and these are pleasant to use on particularly dry skin or areas such as the feet. You may already have a plain emollient at home that can be used, but avoid using a cosmetic body lotion, which may be too highly perfumed for the task. Talcum powder is another medium sometimes used by professionals – for reflexology in particular – and is perfect when applying strokes that do not require much glide.

Preparation

Prepare oils in advance so that you do not interrupt the mood you are trying to create for the massage. The easiest and least messy method of dispensing oil is to keep it in a small flip-top plastic bottle, which will reduce the likelihood of spillage. Alternatively, pour some oil into a small bowl into which you can dip your fingers easily. Most lotions, creams and powders are ready-packaged in suitable containers.

Always warm the oil and your hands before making contact. If possible, place the oil container in hot water or close to a heater for a few minutes before starting the massage.

Application and Contact

The confidence with which you make contact with your partner's skin and apply oil during massage is very important. The aim is for that first touch to feel relaxed and reassuring, transmitting the message that this is the start of the treatment and enabling your partner to get used to your touch. Most professional training teaches that you should not break contact with your partner during a massage, so one hand is placed on them throughout. At home, this may prove difficult at first, especially if you are massaging on the floor. Simply make sure that if you need to break and re-establish contact you do so in a smooth, gentle manner, maintaining the flow of the massage and not leaving your partner wondering whether the treatment has finished. A good massage should have a definite beginning and end so that it feels complete – do not leave your partner with a sense that something was missing.

Applying Oil

1

There are various ways of applying oil. The most obvious is to pour about 2.5ml (½ teaspoon) of oil into the palm of one hand and then rub both palms together to spread the oil evenly. Do not be tempted to wring your hands as you might when washing or applying hand cream, because you want to oil the flat of your hands only. Make sure you apply the oil to your hands slightly away from your partner's body and then gently bring your hands down on to your partner, ready to begin with a long application stroke.

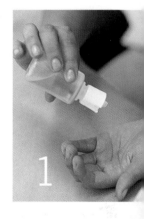

2

The least intrusive way of applying more oil is to leave one hand on your partner's body, slowly pour the oil over the back of the hand and then glide the flat of your other hand across, spreading the oil on the body. A similar method is to turn your contact hand upward and cup it, then pour oil into the palm – this has the added benefit of re-oiling both hands when you glide the other hand over.

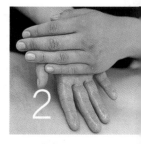

Creating a Relaxed Environment

In later chapters you will see massage being performed in a range of environments, using techniques that are suitable with and without clothing, and working on floor, chair and table. Whichever of these you choose, preparing the surroundings is an important element in creating the atmosphere of comfort and relaxation that is central to any touch therapy.

Warmth

The most important consideration is heating. Body temperature drops while receiving massage, and muscles will not relax in a chilly atmosphere, so the room needs to be warm before the treatment begins. A little fresh air is good, but you should eliminate any draughts. Your partner will really appreciate it if you use warm towels, which can be placed on a radiator or in an airing cupboard ready for use.

Peace and Quiet

The next most important requirement is quiet. You will not relax if there is a television or radio playing in the background or if other members of the family are running in and out of the room. Choose a time when the children are occupied, put the answerphone on, switch off your mobile and give yourself and your partner this gift of time to relax and re-energize.

Having said this, some people like to have music playing, which helps both giver and receiver as they relax into the rhythm of the massage. There are many excellent CDs and cassettes available specifically for this purpose. This idea is not new: centuries ago in Turkey massage often took place close to running water, as listening to its 'music' was considered therapeutic.

Lighting

Avoid direct lighting, as this can feel intrusive and you want your eyes to relax as much as the rest of your body. Depending on the time of day, subdued lights such as table lamps are ideal. Natural light can be good for the daytime, especially the morning, but you may wish to create a special feel in the evening by using candles or oil burners.

Fragrance

Make sure that the room has a pleasant aroma. This can be achieved with flowers, fragrant candles, essential oil burners or incense, but check that your partner likes it, too. Alternatively, simply make sure you have a clean, fresh atmosphere by airing the room earlier in the day. Some people may even prefer quite a clinical environment. The main aim is to create a space in which both of you can relax.

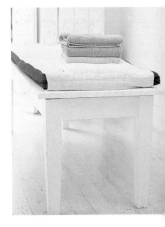

Equipment

Check that you have everything to hand before you start working so that you do not break your concentration.

You will need:

- Your chosen oil
- Box of tissues or kitchen roll
- Two large bath towels or sheets
- Smaller hand towel
- Small cushions or a pillow
- Blanket or lightweight throw if the weather is cold
- Water to drink following the massage

Base of Support

If you are working on the floor, a futon is ideal, but a thick duvet or blankets make excellent substitutes. Make sure that whatever you use has enough space for your partner to be comfortable, plus extra to save your knees when moving around. Do not massage on a bed, as it does not provide the necessary support for the receiver and makes it impossible for you to move easily around his or her body.

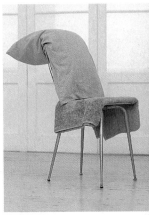

Cover the base with a large towel and use another to cover your partner, only exposing the area of the body you are working on. A small towel can be used to cover a pillow, or rolled up to offer support under the knees or ankles. In general, support the receiver's ankles when they are face down and their knees when they are face up.

If you have a sturdy table that can be adapted to a suitable height, width and length, you can place padding on top and use this as a massage couch. To find the correct height, when standing straight, in the footwear you would be in when giving massage, drop your arms by your side and your knuckles should brush the top of the table. The table should be approximately 1.85m (6ft) long and about 65cm (26in) wide. You will find working on a table much less tiring than working on the floor, and it is easier to manoeuvre around without interrupting the flow of the massage.

If you find yourself massaging regularly, you might wish to invest in a professional couch. Most of these are lightweight, portable and easy to store away, folding up to the size of a large suitcase.

If you are working on a chair, choose one that is sturdy and stable and you will need to use a couple of pillows for comfort and support.

The working positions and posture you should adopt for carrying out the various massage options are described on pages 20–33.

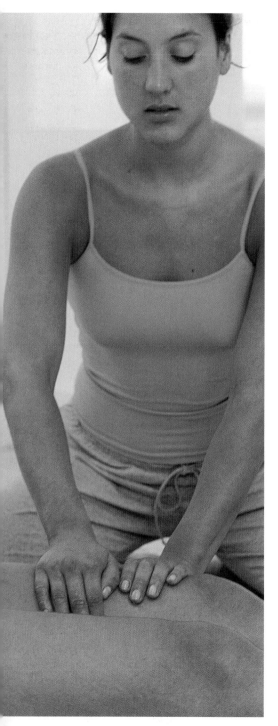

Anatomy

The more that you apply massage, the more you will be able to envisage what lies beneath your hands as they work. This in turn will stimulate your interest in learning about human anatomy and physiology. There are many good introductory books on the subject, but to start you on the path the following pages provide a simple overview.

The human skeleton comprises over 200 bones that have five main functions: support, protection, movement, storage and production.

The muscles also work hard, performing many functions but primarily enabling us to move about, circulate blood, digest and breathe.

Massage can be effective at both superficial and deeper muscle levels: bodywork such as Rolfing claims to work on the muscle fascia (connective tissue) itself. Massage can be used to relax or stimulate, and will also help to disperse knots of muscular spasm and toxins such as lactic acid.

Skeleton

The bones support the body and protect vital organs (as in the ribcage). They make movement possible with lever action at joints and the attachment of muscles. They also store nutrients, and produce red blood cells. Overall, bones are a very industrious body part and should be well cared for with good diet and exercise.

Joints are formed where two or more bones meet. They come in a variety of structures, from immobile links such as those in the skull to free-moving ones like those of the knee and elbow. There is also the ball-and-socket type, as at the shoulder and hip. The movement of free-moving joints is helped along by a lubricant called synovial fluid, which is secreted from a membrane lining a capsule that encases the ends of the bones, rather like oiling a hydraulic piston. Massage stimulates the production of this fluid, which is why sedentary and elderly people find regular treatments really help to sustain their mobility.

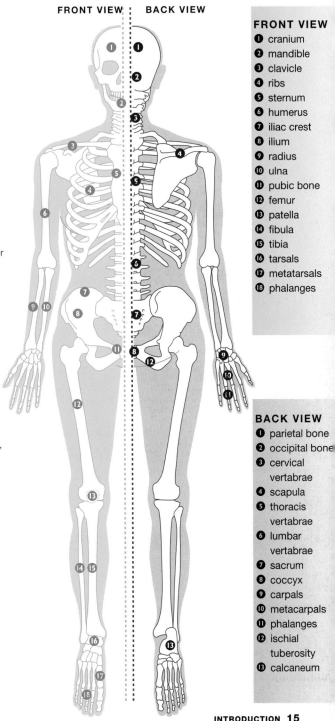

FRONT VIEW **BACK VIEW**

FRONT VIEW

1. sternocleidomastoid
2. deltoid
3. subscapularis
4. pectoralis major
5. serratus anterior
6. biceps
7. abdominals
8. psoas
9. iliacus
10. wrist flexors
11. tensor fascia lata
12. adducters
13. sartorius
14. quadriceps
15. peroneus
16. anterior tibial

BACK VIEW

1. levator scapulae
2. trapezius
3. supraspinatus
4. infraspinatus
5. terus minor
6. terus major
7. rhomboid
8. triceps
9. sacrospinalis
10. latissimus dorsi
11. quadratus lumborum
12. wrist extensors
13. gluteus medius
14. piriformis
15. gluteus maximus
16. gracilis
17. hamstring
18. gastrocnemius
19. soleus

FRONT VIEW **BACK VIEW**

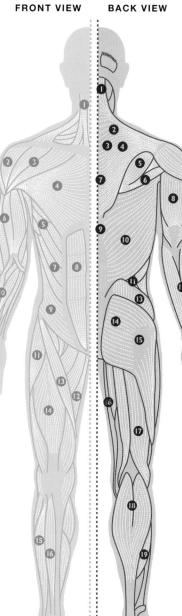

Muscles

There are two main muscle types: those that move automatically, such as the heart, which are called 'involuntary', and those you can move voluntarily with a message from the brain.

The muscles are arranged in layers, symmetrically on each side of the body. Each end is attached to a bone on either side of a joint – these are known as the 'origin' and the 'insertion' of the muscle. Most muscles move in pairs in opposite directions.

Muscles are made up of bundles of fibres or cells, fuelled by blood, lymph and nerves, and encased in fascia (connective tissue): imagine a telephone cable that has an outer casing and a multitude of smaller wires inside, and you will be picturing a muscle. The encased fibres slide between one another when instructed, causing the whole muscle to swell and shorten, which in turn causes the attached bones to move closer together – this process creates body movement. You may have heard the terms 'flexors' and 'extensors' – these are the muscles that, respectively, bend and straighten joints.

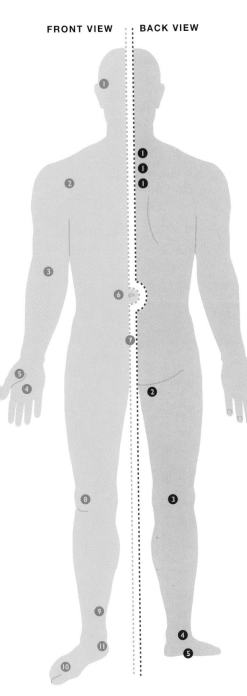

Pressure Points

Pressure points are often used when massaging through clothes. Work on these forms the basis of shiatsu ('finger pressure'), but can equally be incorporated into regular massage as a release mechanism for muscle tension. Working on these points stimulates the nervous system and gives out the signal to relax – rather like acupuncture without the use of needles. Pressure is applied with your thumb pad, although you can also use your elbow when working on the back area.

FRONT VIEW

❶ Side of head and hollows on outside edges of eye sockets *relieves migraine pain*

❷ Hollow at the outer end of the collarbone *stimulates lung function*

❸ Outside of end of elbow crease *relieves arm and shoulder pain and tones large intestine*

❹ Centre of palm *calms emotions and the mind*

❺ Web between thumb and index finger *eliminates colds, toothache and headache*

❻ About 7cm (3in) to either side of navel *relaxes stomach tension and aids digestion*

❼ Below navel, deep pressure with four flat fingers *stimulates whole body*

❽ Top of shinbone, in curve toward knee, *encourages well-being and energizes*

❾ Above inner ankle bone, four fingers up, *relieves menstrual pains*

❿ Between big toe and second toe, 3–5cm (1¼–2in) above join, *stabilizes liver function*

⓫ Inside heel at centre *stimulates kidneys*

BACK VIEW

❶ Either side of spine *brings equilibrium to body functions*

❷ Side of buttocks *relieves menstrual problems and relaxes pelvis*

❸ Back of knee (well supported) *relieves sciatica*

❹ Either side of Achilles tendon *stimulates water flow and relieves lower back pain*

❺ Under ball of foot *calms and relaxes generally*

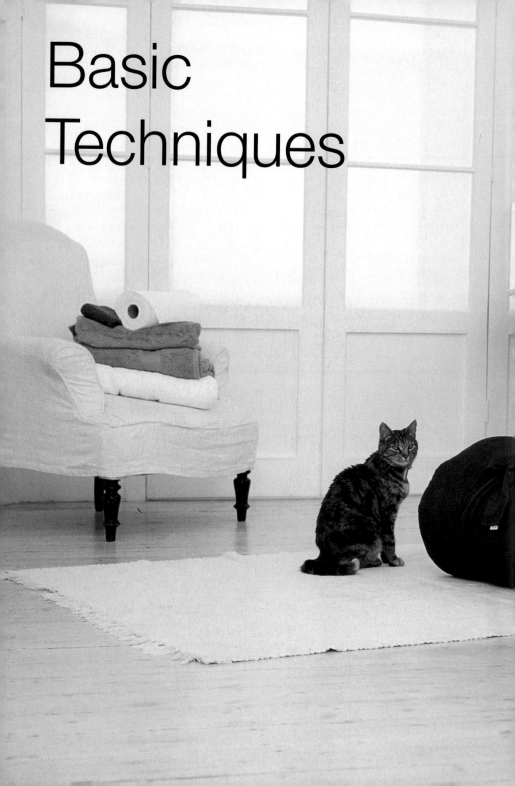

Basic Techniques

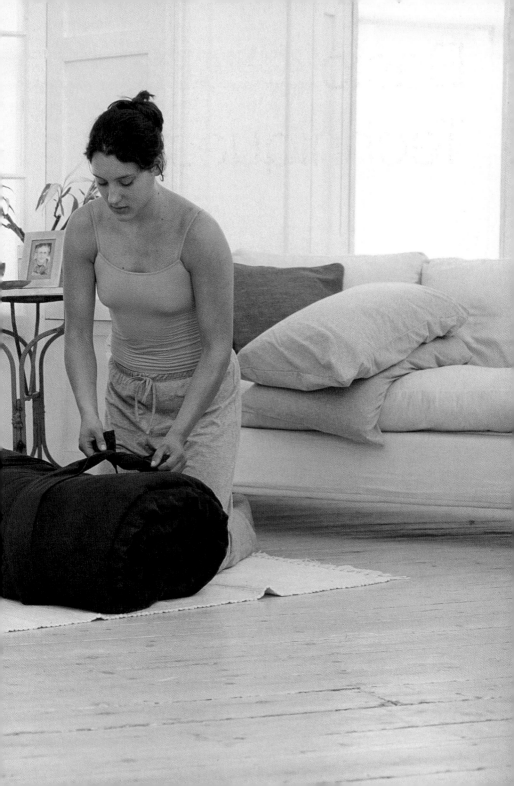

Giving Massage

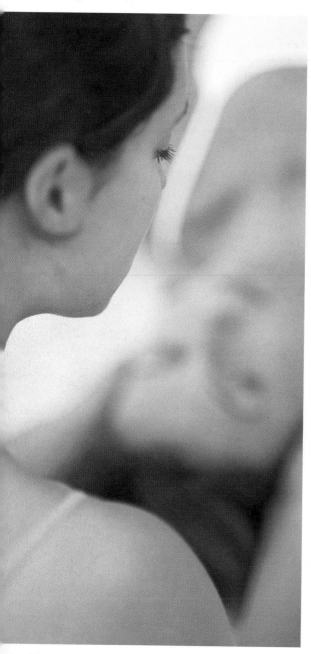

The techniques covered in this book are the 'mother' strokes of massage that are practised in the Western hemisphere. Known as Swedish Massage, they consist of effleurage (stroking), petrissage (squeezing), percussion (tapotement), friction and stretching.

These movements can be applied at different speeds and levels of pressure. The most important keys to a good massage are the rhythm and flow, so try to develop this sense and eventually you will not have to think about every stroke you are applying – they will come naturally.

In order for your partner to feel the benefits of a massage, the various strokes need to be applied in a specific order:

- 'making contact'
- effleurage
- petrissage, percussion and friction
- some stretching, more effleurage and a 'holding' or 'grounding' technique

In general, massage strokes are applied working toward the heart. For example, if you are working on the legs you will apply firmer pressure on the upward stroke and lighter pressure on the return stroke.

The procedure for a whole

body massage is as follows. With your partner lying face down, make the contact stroke by placing the flat of your hand confidently, and with good pressure, on the sacrum (see page 15), then, using the strokes described in the following pages, work over the whole of the back area, including the top of the buttocks and the lower back, the shoulder blades and the upper back, and, lastly, the sides of the torso. Do not apply pressure directly to the spine: work on either side of it.

Move to the legs, working up from the ankle (reducing pressure over the back of the knee) to the top and return, finishing on the foot.

Turn your partner over and begin with the shoulders, working on the back and front simultaneously. Move from the neck up to the scalp, then to the face. Next, massage each arm separately, working up the limb and returning, to finish with the wrist and hand. Next move to the ribcage, the sides of the torso and abdomen. Finish with the legs, again working up from the ankle (avoiding pressure on the knee) to the top and returning, to finish on the foot.

Just as you start any massage with 'contact', you should end with 'connecting' or 'grounding' holds. Either rest your hands on each foot with your thumbs placed on the instep area and apply medium pressure, or place your hands on two separate parts of the body.

A whole body massage should take 1–1½ hours, but as you become proficient you may wish to concentrate on areas of tension or give short remedial treatments.

MASSAGE AREAS

A whole body massage is usually broken down into seven distinct areas.

Back
- torso
- legs and feet

Front
- neck and shoulders
- scalp and face
- arms and hands
- torso
- legs and feet

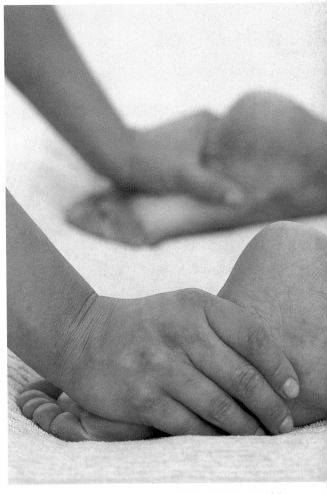

Posture and Position

Whether you are working with the receiver on a chair, the floor or a table, your own posture and position play an important part in the treatment by ensuring good control of rhythm, flow and pressure. Your posture and position also need to be correct in order to avoid mechanical stress on your own body.

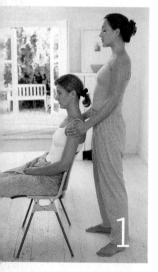

Chair

Some massage techniques can be carried out with the receiver seated. This is useful during pregnancy or for the elderly, and is also suitable for massage in an office.

receiver: There are several positions that the receiver can adopt for chair work:

- Sitting astride a chair, leaning forward into pillows, and resting her forearms and head on the chairback.
- Sitting on a chair and leaning forward onto a table or desk with a cushion for support.
- Sitting upright in a chair when you are massaging the head, neck and shoulders from behind or the limbs from the front.

giver: In the upright posture (1), stand with your back straight, feet slightly apart and body weight balanced equally on both legs. In the 'warrior' position (2), stand with your legs parallel but with one foot ahead of the other, toes facing forward to provide a stable base. As you lean forward, raise the heel of the back leg slightly and keep the front leg relaxed. Your arms should be straight or flexed slightly and your back more or less straight.

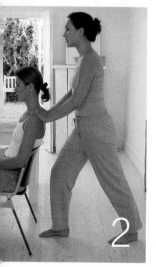

Floor

A futon makes an ideal support for the receiver; otherwise, use a duvet, blankets or anything else suitable to provide some padding.

Make sure you have enough space in which to move around easily without interrupting the flow of the treatment.

The main rules of posture for floor work are to:

- Relax your shoulders and upper back.
- Move from the hips and legs.
- As far as possible, keep your spine straight.
- Breathe!

To work at the top of the receiver's body, kneel either side of her head so your knees are parallel to her ears. From here, you can lean straight forward over the point of contact, or straight back for stretches.

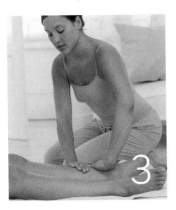
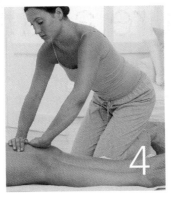

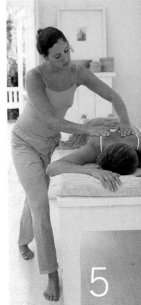

When working on areas such as the calves, thighs and sides of the torso, kneel side-on to your partner (3), with your knees apart and shoulders relaxed.

As you stretch forward, rise up slightly on your knees, moving from your hips and keeping your back and arms as straight as possible (4). Release on the return stroke. For long, sweeping strokes up the legs or back, position yourself to one side of your partner, knees together and sitting back on your heels. To work on the feet or for 'grounding' at the end of a treatment, adopt the side-on position (see 3).

Table

Using a table (see page 13 for dimensions) places less strain on your back and is not as physically demanding as working on the floor. You will also find it easier to move around.

The main rules for working on a table are:

- Stand square to the table.
- Bend from your knees and hips.
- Do not twist your body.

When working at either end of the table use the upright posture or the warrior position. The latter can also be used when working side-on.

The 'lunge' posture (5) is also used to either side of the table for applying long strokes without having to bend your back. Lean against the table or position yourself slightly away from it. Keep both feet flat on the floor, then, as you move forward, flex the front knee and keep the back leg straight. Keep your arms straight for even pressure.

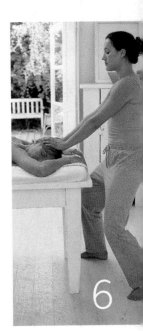

The 'monkey' position (6) is used when pressure needs to move from one hand to the other and when strokes move from side to side rather than up and back. Standing slightly away from the table, place your body weight equally over both feet, with your knees slightly flexed and your back and arms straight. Shift your weight from one foot to the other to produce a side-to-side movement.

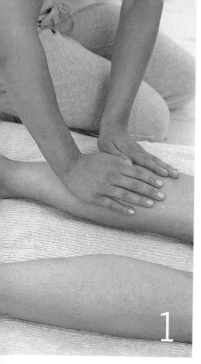

Effleurage

A French word meaning 'stroking', effleurage is the simplest technique to perform and can be used everywhere on the body. It is a rhythmic movement, which is used especially to:

- Make and break contact.
- Enable your partner to relax under your touch.
- Enable you to sense areas of tension.
- Spread massage oil, lotion, cream or talcum powder easily.
- Connect different parts of the body.
- Warm the muscles in preparation for deeper work.

Effleurage also helps to improve blood and lymph flows and induces relaxation. In particular, it is the main stroke used to bring out the aromatherapeutic benefits of essential oils.

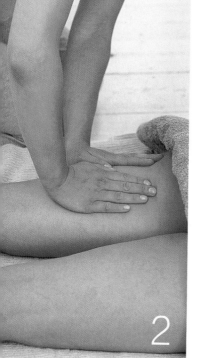

Flat-handed

Oil the flat of your hands and, with your fingers together and wrists relaxed, make contact with your partner and glide both hands simultaneously (1) with pressure and momentum upward to your natural reach (2), then separate and return along the sides of the limb or torso in a breaststroke-like movement. Repeat several times. Remember to reduce the pressure over joint areas, and when working on the back place your hands on either side of the spine – do not work directly on it. Another way of administering this stroke on the back area is to make broad, circular movements, spiralling up to the shoulders and returning flat-handed down the sides.

For extra pressure, one hand can be placed on top of the other to administer the stroke – this is known as 'double-handed' or 'reinforced' effleurage. Pressure can also be applied by the thumb only.

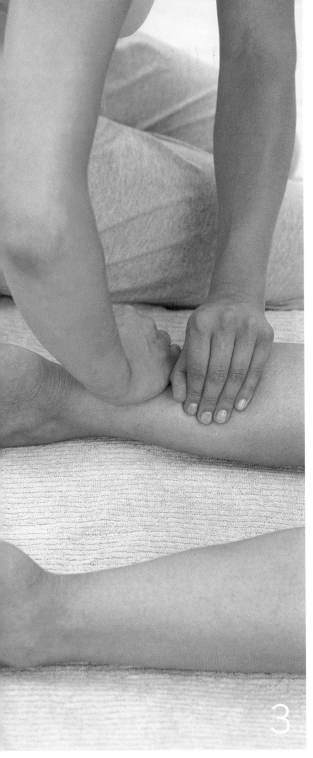

Cupped

This variation, in which the hands are cupped and horizontal, one in front of the other, is especially useful when you are working on the legs and arms. Oil your hands, then make contact with your partner (3) and glide up the limb to your natural reach (4), turn and use the flat-handed stroke to return. Cupped effleurage is a very soothing stroke for the calf and arm muscles, which are often very sensitive areas. When working on the upper thigh, take the stroke further with the outside hand, turning the inside hand discreetly on your partner's inner thigh so as not to be intrusive.

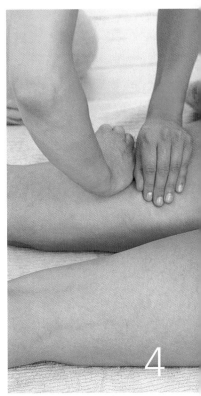

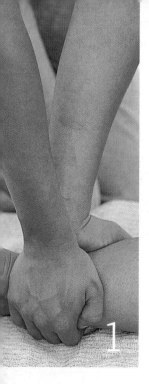

Petrissage

Petrissage is the general name given to any stroke that presses, squeezes and rolls the muscles under the skin. It also includes kneading and wringing techniques. This is a medium-depth stroke that is used after effleurage, and it acts to:

- 'Milk' the muscles of waste products, literally squeezing the tension, toxins and tiredness out of the body.
- Prepare for deeper work, such as friction (see page 30).
- Break up specific knots of tension.
- Stretch and loosen muscle fibres and fascia (connective tissue).
- Stimulate circulation to an area.

Petrissage also helps the blood and oxygen return, and to relax the muscles.

Mirrored Hands

With your hands on top of the muscle and supporting the underside with your fingertips, squeeze the heels of your hands downward, each hand mirroring the other (1). Then bring your fingers upward so that you have a handful of flesh between the two. Slide the heel of your hands back and repeat in a continuous rhythm of squeezing and releasing, working upward over the muscle.

Alternate Hands

Using the same procedure, you can work your hands alternately – one hand squeezing downward and stretching upward, followed by the other (2). On a larger area, such as the sides of the buttocks, this is particularly useful for working on one side at a time.

One-handed Petrissage

This technique is most effective when strong pressure is required or when you are working on your partner's shoulders or along their back on either side of the spine. With one hand resting on the limb or torso, repeat the petrissage with the other, sweeping over the muscle and adjusting the pressure according to your partner's tension.

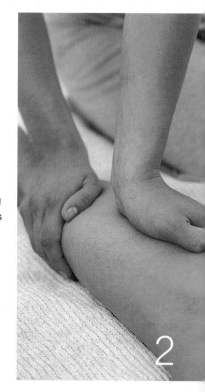

Other Petrissage Techniques

Wringing

This is a stroke that literally 'wrings' out the tension and toxins stored in muscles (3). Using the whole of your hand with the thumb close to the fingers, work alternately backward and forward in a continuous flow, lifting the skin toward you with one hand and pushing it away with the other. Wringing is mostly used on the calf and thigh, but if you are working on small muscles you can open your thumbs wide to get a firm grip as you wring.

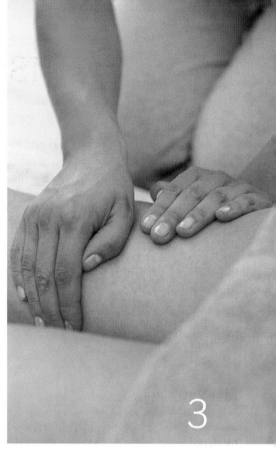

Kneading

Kneading, often mistaken as the only stroke of petrissage, requires medium pressure and should be applied only after the muscle has been relaxed, usually over large, fleshy areas. The slower and deeper the stroke, the more beneficial it is. Using the whole of your hands with the thumbs spread (4), lean them firmly into the muscle and use them alternately, working them toward each other, squeezing and rolling the muscle in a side-to-side action – imagine you are kneading dough. Work your way up the muscle, keeping contact with both hands in a continuous, rhythmic motion.

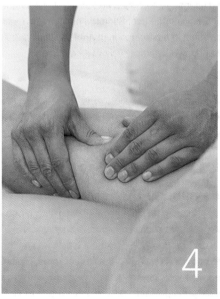

Percussion

SAFETY FIRST

Take care when using percussive strokes, because they are not suitable for bony areas, the spine, head and neck, or the back of the knee. Nor should they be used where there is any inflammation, strain, paralysed muscle or varicose veins, or in the kidney area.

Percussion, named after the noise it makes, is known by professionals as tapotement, the French word for 'light tapping'. It consists of brisk strokes made by using both hands alternately in a rhythmic motion. As with the percussion section of an orchestra, the strokes build up slowly to a crescendo and then end abruptly.

The technique is used to:

- Improve local circulation.
- Tone and stimulate soft tissue areas, such as the outer thighs and buttocks.
- Stimulate nerve endings.

No oils or creams are necessary.

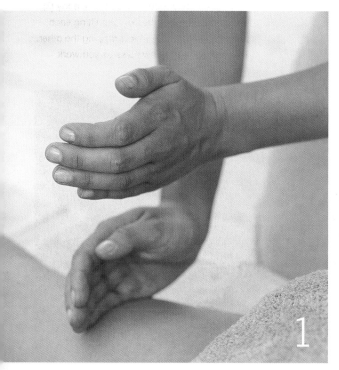

Hacking

Make sure your hands and wrists are relaxed by stroking and shaking them. In a chopping movement and with a flick of the wrists, bring your hands down alternately 4–5cm (1½–2in) apart onto your partner's body surface (1). Only the little finger should hit the tissue, with the other fingers cascading onto it. The first hand then rises rapidly as the other hand descends. It may take a little practice to develop a smooth rhythm – try working in time to music with a good drumbeat. Once you are proficient, you can vary the pace and strength of hacking according to your partner's requirements. A heavier hacking stroke can be applied with your fingers curled and closed together. Always keep your shoulders and elbows relaxed when doing this stroke.

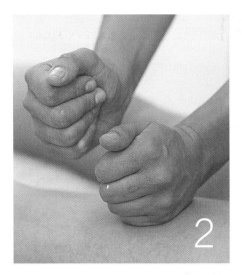

Pummelling

Lightweight pummelling – or pounding, as it is sometimes called – is performed (in the same way as other percussive strokes) with a flick of the wrist. For heavier work, the wrist is locked and the elbow bent, lowering the forearm and thereby providing more body weight behind the stroke. Make your hands into loose fists with your thumbs on top, then bring them down alternately (2), as in hacking, with the fleshy (palmar) side bouncing firmly on the tissue and making a strong, rhythmic beating sound. This stroke is usually applied only to large, well-padded areas of muscle such as the buttocks and thighs.

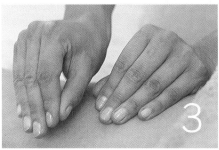

Cupping

Make a cup shape with your hands, keeping your fingers straight. Moving from your forearm, not your wrist, bring your hands down alternately onto your partner's body (3), trapping air against the skin and lifting each hand 4–5cm (1½–2in) while dropping the other. This will make a hollow noise as you work across the area.

Flicking

This technique is sometimes called plucking. With straight fingers, bring your thumbs and fingertips down onto your partner's skin and, in a quick action, take up a small piece of flesh (4) and then let it slip easily away with each stroke, turning your wrist very slightly as you release. Alternate your hands in a steady, rhythmic motion.

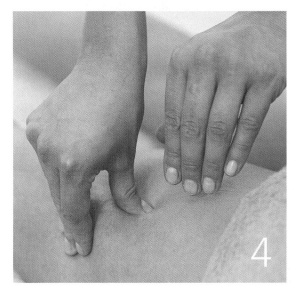

Friction

Take care when using friction,
and do not apply if the nerve
is inflamed or on any area
that reacts with a protective
contraction.
In particular, friction must be
carried out gently and
stopped immediately if nerve
pain is exacerbated, as it
will be counterproductive
to overstep the mark.

A deep and focused stroke, friction is carried out after effleurage and petrissage. The stroke uses mainly the fingertips, thumbs and heel of the hands, and is often done with only one hand at a time and with little or no gliding, so that oils and creams are rarely needed. The movements reach deep down into the tissue where more tensions may be hidden.

Friction is used to:

- Reduce oedema (water retention).
- Stretch and release knots of tension.
- Disperse calcifications around joint areas, e.g. as in gout.
- Stimulate the digestive tract and colon.
- Treat intense, intermittent pain from branches of the main nervous system.

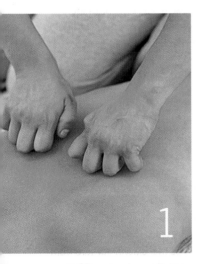

Straight Knuckling

Curl your hands into loose fists and, with your knuckles flat on your partner's skin, glide up the leg or back using the middle section of your fingers (1). Do not rotate your fingers and always work toward the heart to aid blood and lymph flows. This stroke works deep into the muscle and tissue to release stubborn tensions and deposits.

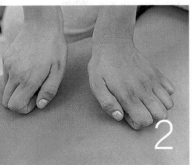

Circular Knuckling

As with straight knuckling, curl your hands into a loose fist, but instead of straight gliding, rotate the fingers at the same time to make a circular movement (2). Performed lightly, this relaxes the chest and shoulder areas, and you can also use it to work deep into the pectoral muscles or around the shoulder blade to release long-standing tensions. This stroke is very pleasant to receive on the backs of the hands and the feet.

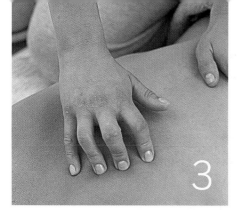

Circular Friction

Work with one hand at a time, resting the other on your partner for reassurance (3). With your fingers slightly apart, apply even pressure through your fingertips by moving the tissues over the body's structure in a small, circular movement that starts gently and increases progressively. You can also work your fingertips backward and forward.

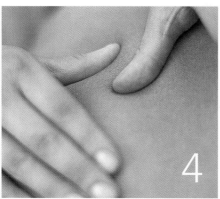

Thumb Rolling

Using the length of your thumbs and leaning into your partner's skin with your whole body weight, bring one thumb down behind the other, pushing away with short, deep strokes in a rhythmic motion (4). This stroke can be applied on any area to smooth out knotty muscle fibres, and it is especially useful in releasing tension between the spine and shoulder blades.

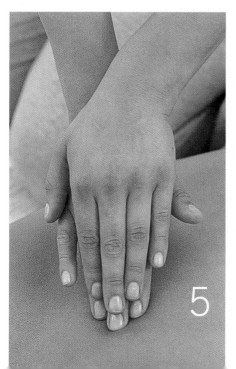

Circling

Place one hand on top of the other with your fingers straight but relaxed. Lean into the muscle with your fingertips and slowly make tiny circles, working around the joints and areas of tension (5). The aim is to move the underlying tissue rather than glide over the skin's surface. On the back, work on the nerves and muscles that extend outward from the spine, never over the spine itself. When circling the knee, use your thumbs rather than your fingertips.

Completing the Massage

At the end of a massage treatment your partner will be feeling somewhat distant and relaxed, so it is very important to finish in a sensitive manner by bringing their awareness back slowly. Always finish with a grounding stroke to complete the routine and encourage your partner to stay still and rest for a few minutes before slowly getting up.

Feathering

This stroke is used to soothe and calm when completing a massage sequence, leaving your partner relaxed. Keeping your arms and hands relaxed, stroke your partner's skin lightly downward (1), using one hand after the other and covering the maximum area without changing position. With each stroke lighten the contact until you are feathering slightly above the skin.

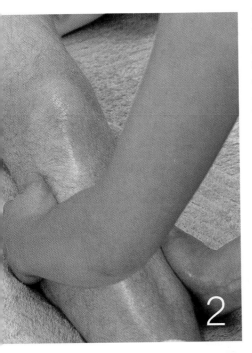

Rocking

This light pressure stroke is used after working on a particular area of the body, or early in the massage to relax and loosen the limbs, encouraging your partner's body to let go and succumb to the treatment. When working on the arms, get your partner to lie face up and support the upper arm by cupping your hands on either side. Rock the arm back and forth between your hands, slowly moving down the arm and increasing the pace around the wrist area. Finish by stroking over the fingers. Repeat on the opposite arm.

To rock the legs, get your partner to lie face up. Place your hands on either side of the thigh, rock the leg back and forth between your hands, moving slowly down the leg, and finish by stroking over the toes. Repeat on the opposite leg. If you are at the end of a massage treatment, end by grounding your partner (see step 3).

Grounding

To ground your partner at the end of the massage, place your thumbs on her insteps and the webs and palms of your hand on the fronts or soles of her feet (3), employing a strong, even pressure for at least 30 seconds. If you have been working on the upper body only, grounding will also help to 'reconnect' the receiver, completing the massage in a caring way and indicating to your partner that this is the end of the treatment.

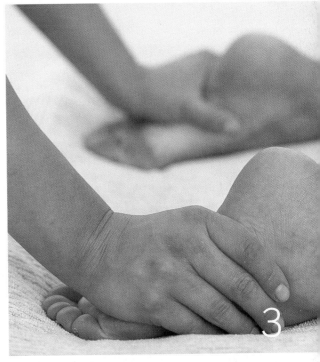

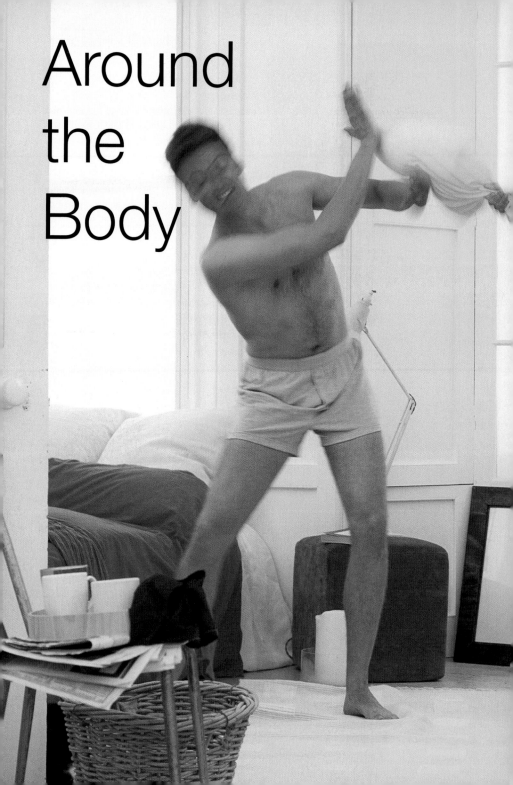

Around the Body

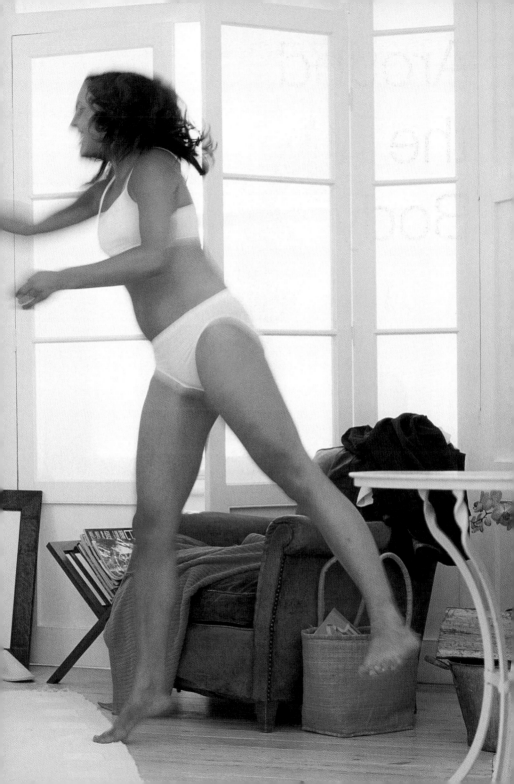

Energizing Morning Massage

Many people think that massage is just for relaxing and is ideal before bedtime, but it can in fact be used at all times of the day and be either stimulating or relaxing. In order to get all your systems moving in the morning, strokes such as percussion and friction are used to stimulate the blood and lymph flows, ready for the day's action.

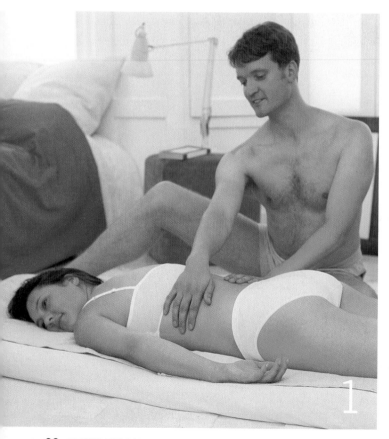

1

With your partner lying face down, position yourself side-on and with both hands apply wringing strokes (see page 27) across the whole back. Place one hand on the side of the back nearest to you and the other on the far side. Push forward with the heel of the nearside hand while pulling back with the fingers of the other, working in a continual criss-cross movement.

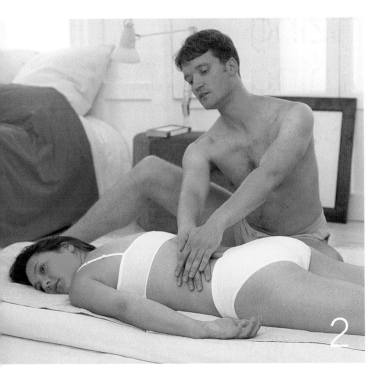

2

With one hand palm down on your partner's back, place your other hand on top and, using double-handed effleurage strokes (see page 24), glide in large, circular movements over the whole of the back.

3

Using flicking movements (see page 29), work all over the shoulder blade area, avoiding the spine. This will stimulate the circulation and help to clear the lungs of any congestion.

SAFETY FIRST

Remember: always work on either side of the spine, never directly over it.

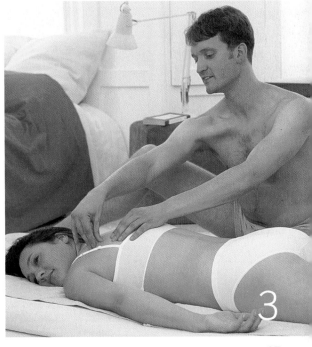

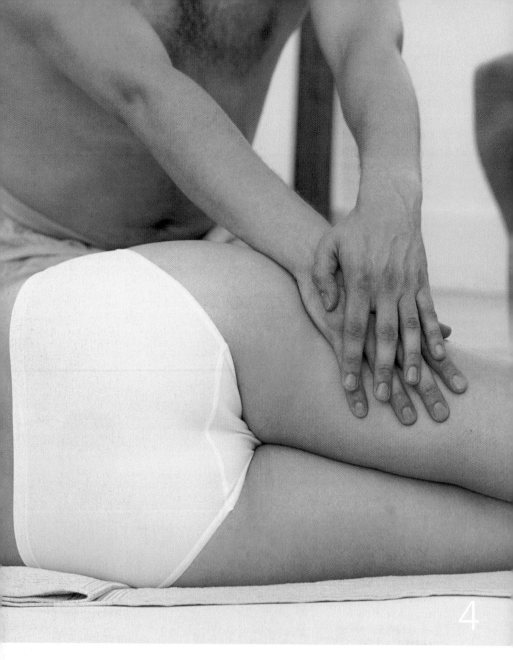

4

4

With your partner lying comfortably on their side, use
double-handed effleurage strokes to massage over the
whole of the back of the upper leg and thigh.

5

With your partner in the same position, and making sure that the leg is supported, use wringing strokes to work over the top of the leg between the knee and the hip.

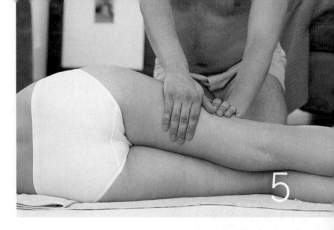

6

Make your hands into loose fists and lightly pummel the fleshy sides up and down the thigh alternately (see page 29).

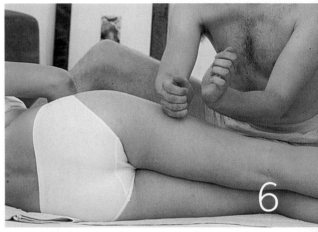

7

After completing the pummelling, uncurl your fingers and shake your hands to relax them. Lightly bring down the edge of each hand alternately in hacking strokes (see page 28), slowly gathering momentum. Once you have established a good, sustainable rhythm, work on the muscle directly.

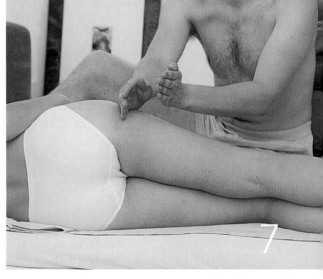

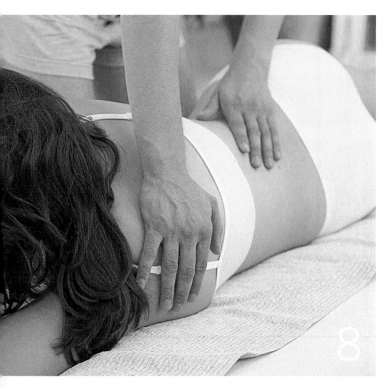

8

Place one hand on your partner's far shoulder and the other on the nearer lower back. Push forward with the heel of the hand on the shoulder, at the same time pulling back with the fingers on the lower back, creating a long stretch diagonally across the length of the torso. Get your partner to roll onto her other side, switch to her other side, and switching hands repeat the stretch.

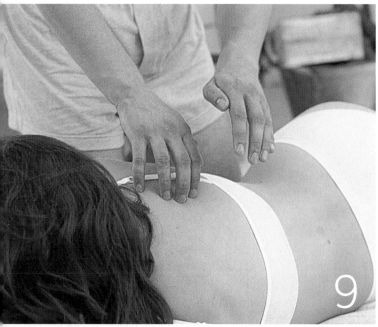

9

Using the tops of your fingers in rotation, drum gently on your partner's skin raising each finger before the next touches. Use both hands simultaneously and increase the speed but not the pressure. Using this drumming motion, work over the muscles between the shoulder blade and the spine to relieve any congestion in the lung area.

10

This is another variation on hacking (see page 28), called 'open-handed hacking'. The fingers are spread apart to give a lighter pressure and sensation. Using this stroke, work all over the back area, avoiding the spine, to stimulate blood circulation and to get everything moving for the day ahead.

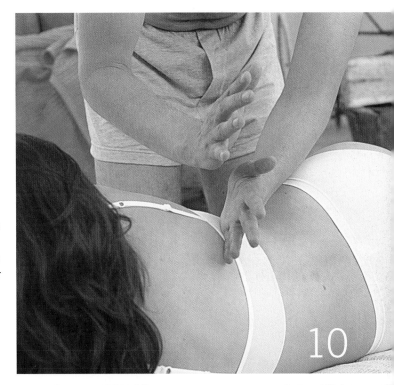

11

This dynamic use of hacking is taken from Indian Ayurvedic massage, in which it is applied to the head. Work lightly over the whole of your partner's scalp to stimulate blood flow. This technique is also extremely beneficial in encouraging hair growth and condition.

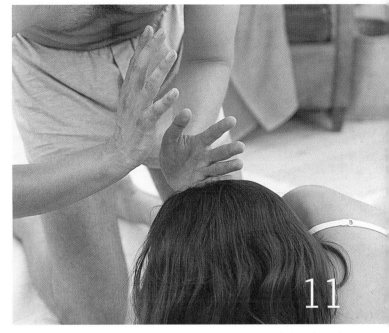

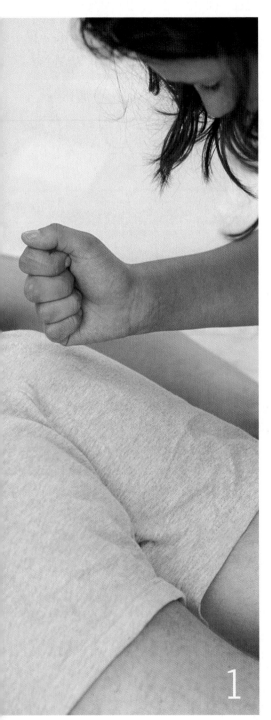

Lymphatic Massage

Applied in the mornings, lymphatic massage will give your immune system a boost and encourage the elimination of toxins and waste products, leaving you feeling more energetic and focused. Your lymphatic system plays an important part in maintaining correct fluid levels and defending the body against disease. It is a complicated filtering system made up of tiny vessels, and the lymph glands have no muscles to help the flow and drainage, so massage achieves this manually and will speed up a sluggish system.

1

With your partner lying face down, make a fist with your right hand, swing out and firmly but not painfully punch the right buttock with your fist.

Repeat five times.

Repeat on the opposite side.

2

With your wrist loose, use the back of your hand to pat the kidneys very gently.

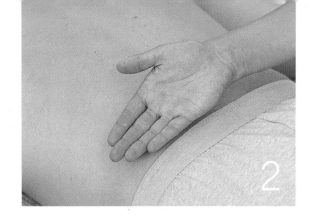

3

Make a fist with your hand, ask your partner to take a deep breath and, on the out breath, thump the back below the shoulder blades on either side of the spine.

Repeat five times.

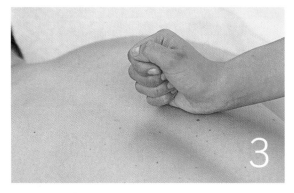

4

Supporting your partner's arm at the wrist and upper arm, lift it upward and then release it, at the same time leaning back slightly to give a gentle pull.

Repeat several times before moving to the opposite side.

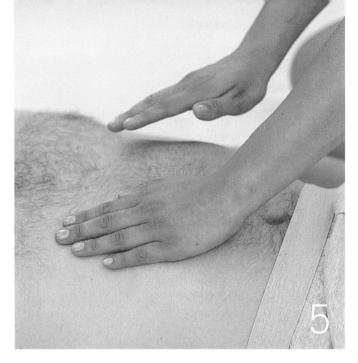

5

Ask your partner to turn face up and take a deep breath. On the out breath, slap the ribcage lightly and quickly with the palms of both hands for 30 seconds.

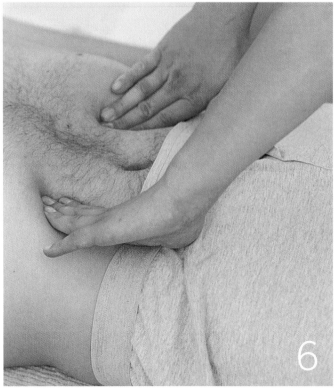

6

Moving your hands to below your partner's ribcage, massage firmly from the sides of the body inward toward the navel.

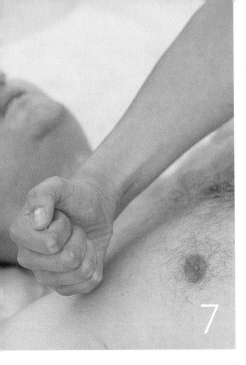

7

Ask your partner to take a deep breath and on the out breath, using your right hand in a fist, thump the area under the collarbone five times in succession.

8

Repeat step 7 but use your left hand to clear the heart lymphatics on the right side of your partner's body.

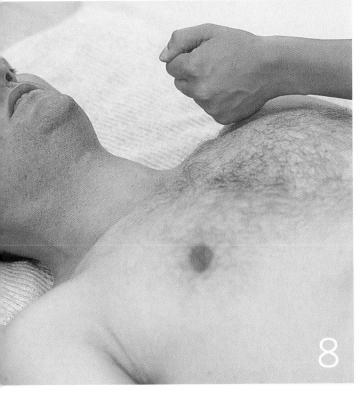

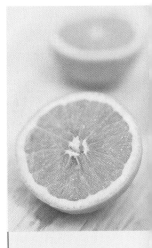

Tip

A glass of hot water and a slice of lemon, grapefruit or orange is a refreshing, cleansing and stimulating start to the day.

9

Place the flat of your hand on the breast bone between the nipples, ask your partner to take a deep breath and, on the out breath, thump the top of your hand with the fist of the other hand five times.

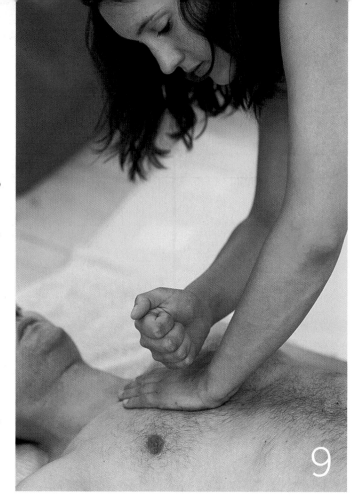

9

10

Using the tips of your fingers in a tapping motion, work across the top of the chest very lightly.

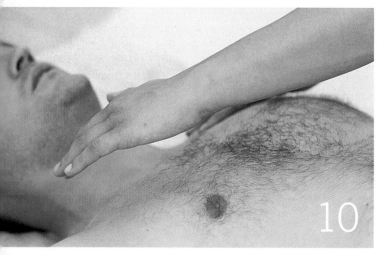

10

11

Again using the tips of the fingers, tap down the sides of the neck simultaneously.

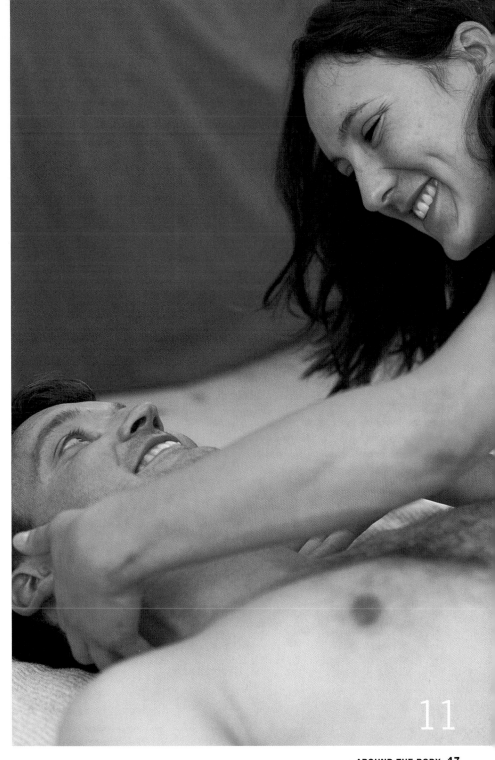

11

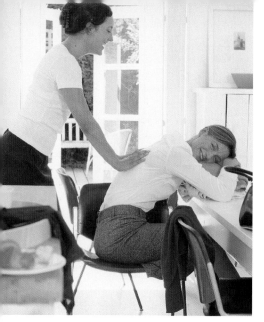

Neck and Upper Back

This is an easy routine that you can do sitting at a kitchen table, desk or any other stable surface at a suitable height. Make your partner comfortable, with her arms and upper body cushioned.

1

Rest your right hand on your partner's right shoulder to make contact. Using your left hand, work from the left of the spine outward, applying steady pressure from the heel of the hand and slowly moving from the lower back up to the top of the shoulder blade.

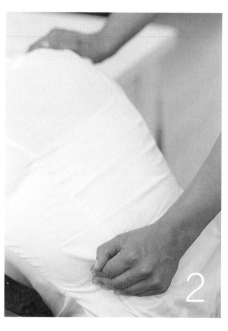

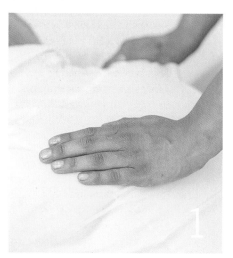

2

Make a fist and effleurage (see page 24) in large circles, always applying the pressure on the upward strokes toward the heart.

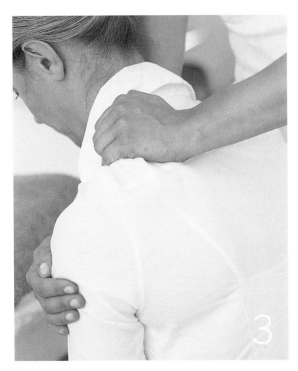

3

Move side-on to your partner, bring her upright and move your right hand from the right shoulder across to her upper left arm, giving support across the front of the upper torso. With your left hand, lift and squeeze the muscle between her left shoulder blade and spine with the heel of your hand and fingers.

Move to the other side and repeat steps 1–3.

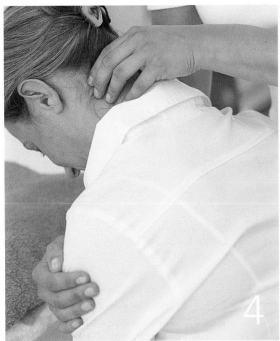

4

Ask your partner to drop her head slightly and, still supporting the front of her shoulders, squeeze the muscles of the neck between your fingers and thumb, working up toward the base of the skull. If you are finishing the massage here, 'ground' your partner by gently squeezing down the arms and legs, and hold her feet for ten seconds.

SAFETY FIRST

Remember: always work on either side of the spine, never directly over it.

Upper Arms and Shoulders

After a long day at work tension appears in the muscles that stabilize the shoulder.

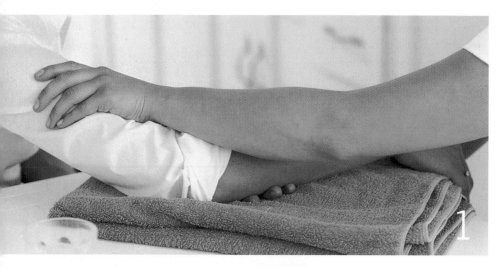

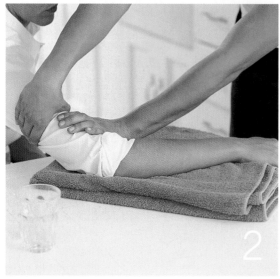

1

With one hand under your partner's elbow for support, effleurage (see page 24) the upper arm from elbow to shoulder, turning your hand at the top and returning down the outside of the arm.

2

Turning side on to your partner, wring (see page 27) the muscles of the upper arm, using continuous, rhythmic strokes and covering the whole of the area.

3

Glide upward from the wrist to the shoulder, applying pressure with your thumb pads, tracing the contours as you go.

Repeat three to five times.

4

With one hand supporting the upper arm and the other holding your partner's hand firmly, lean back and give a comfortable stretch to your partner's arm and shoulder. Hold for five to ten seconds and then release slowly.

Move to the other arm and repeat steps 1–4.

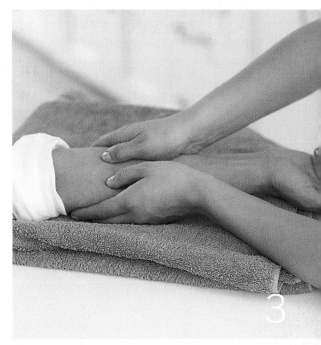

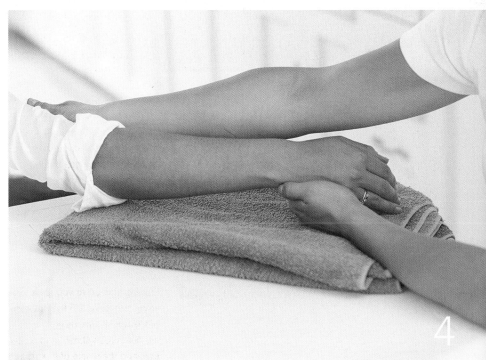

Back

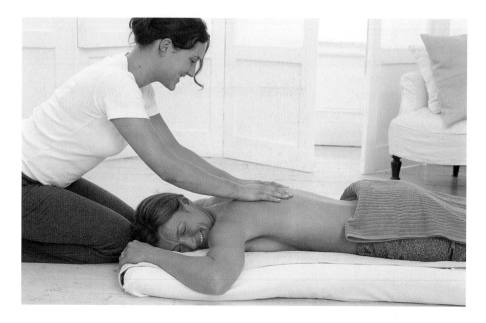

Back pain accounts for more lost working days than any other complaint. The back is vulnerable because it is our main supportive structure and it stores enormous amounts of tension in the large muscles that cover the area. The majority of people visiting a massage therapist will have backache of some kind, usually due to poor posture habits.

The back is the largest single area you will be massaging, and it is often the best place to start a routine, as it enables your partner to relax. Make sure that you are comfortable and reserve your energy by moving your body from the hips rather than just your arms and upper body. You can add the back routine to others that treat the head or legs and buttocks, but it is just as effective on its own.

Position yourself at your partner's head with her arms placed out to the sides. With warm hands and warmed oil, make contact by gently placing your hands on her shoulder blades and hold for ten to twenty seconds. You may observe some tightness and rigidity or even see the muscles twitching as they start to relax.

1

Using flat-handed effleurage (see page 24), work on either side of the spine, gliding your hands downward to the lower back. If you are working on the floor, you may find it necessary to rise up on your knees to drop your weight behind the stroke as you stretch forward toward the lower back area.

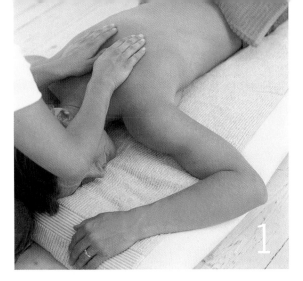

2

At the lower back, glide both hands out to the sides of the torso and then bring them up the sides with a slight pull, ending level with her armpits.

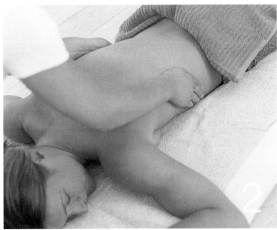

3

Bring your hands inward toward the spine, gliding over the tops of the shoulder blades.

At this stage you can either repeat steps 1–3 four or five times or continue with the sequence.

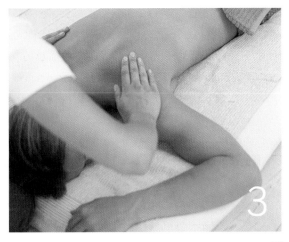

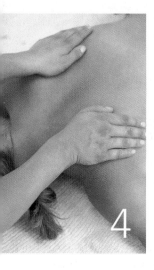

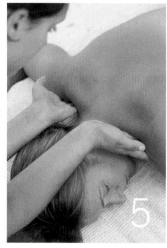

4 & 5

At the shoulder blades turn your hands outward and bring them over the top of the shoulders, so that the flats of your hands are now turned upward with the fingers resting on the front of the shoulders. Scoop your hands inward toward the neck.

Repeat steps 1–5 three or four times. On the final stroke, you may wish to bring your hands up the neck, finishing at the hairline.

Reverse Effleurage

This part of the routine is called 'reverse effleurage', as you are working in the opposite direction to before. It is a potentially deeper treatment and concentrates on the upper back and shoulder area where tension, discomfort and even pain are often experienced. To work more deeply and break down tension in the area, a variety of strokes can be used after step 3 (see page 53). These are effective in stretching tight muscles and breaking down knots of tension, and at the same time promote relaxation and circulation in the area.

Place your thumbs flat on either side of the spine and, using effleurage, glide both thumbs simultaneously downward to the lower back. You may feel nodules and observe a change of skin tone in particularly tense areas.

Repeat three or four times.

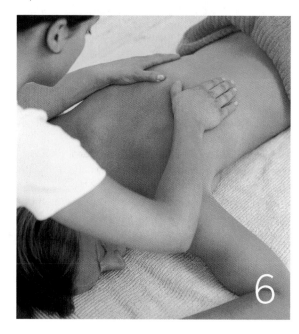

7

In the triangle between the spine, the edge of the shoulder blade and the base of the neck, and working first on one side and then the other, apply thumb rolls (see page 31), making sure that you use the entire length of your thumbs and not just the pads. Where you come across knots of tension, spend a little time working on the area and then soothe with lighter, broader strokes.

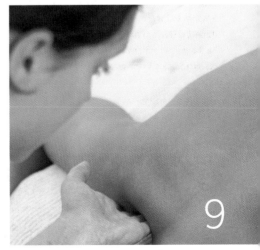

8

Make sure that your partner's head is facing away. Rest one hand on the upper back and with the other make a fist with your fingers. Using only the flat part of the fist, not the knuckles, glide outward from the base of the neck to the edge of the shoulder, keeping it flat to the surface. Ease off the pressure at the end of the stroke, lift the hand and return to the base of the neck. Adjust the pressure in response to the tightness of the muscle. This is called 'du poing' effleurage and is used for tight or highly developed muscles.

Repeat three or four times and change sides.

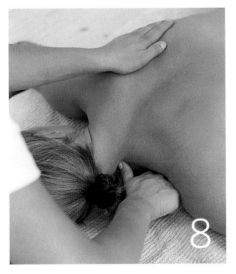

9

Hold and support your partner's head, which should be turned away. With the web of your hand, glide down the neck with the palm and fingers on the underside, applying gentle pressure and pushing outward, ending at the top of the arm. Repeat a few times before moving to the other side. If you feel confident, at the same time try moving your partner's head slightly to the opposite side, which applies a very gentle stretch to the muscles and helps to release tension. Do not do this if your partner suffers from osteoporosis or spondylosis (inflammation of the vertabrae).

Self-massage

One of the best ways of combating stress and repetitive strain injury (see page 112) is to take regular breaks during your working day. Here is a simple routine you can do while you are at work. Repeat each movement as many times as you need in the time you have – whether you spend five minutes or twenty minutes working on yourself, you will feel the benefit and have more energy for the rest of the day. This routine is particularly good for neck tension, which often causes headaches or stiffness.

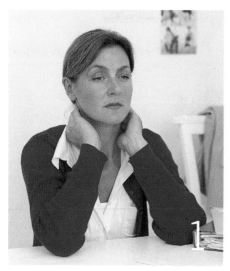

1

Resting your elbows on the desk, place your fingers at the back of your neck behind your ears, leaning your head forward slightly. Make sure you are comfortable, and then with the pads of your fingers work down the length of your neck on either side of the vertebrae by rotating your fingers and applying pressure.

2

Place one hand on the desk and the other on the opposite shoulder. Tilting your head slightly away from the area you are massaging, squeeze the muscle between the fingers and heel of your hand, working from the base of the neck to the edge of the shoulder.

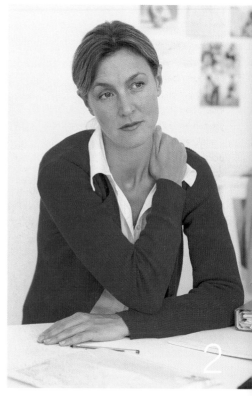

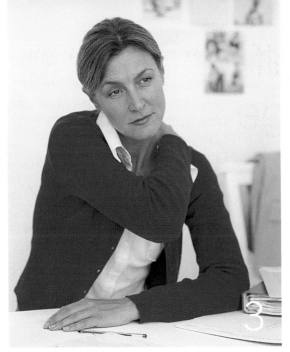

3

In the same position as for step 2, place your fingers on the top of your shoulder muscle and rotate your finger pads while applying pressure, again working from the base of the neck to the edge of your shoulder.

Move to the other side and repeat steps 2 and 3.

4

To complete the massage, take your ear lobes between your thumbs and index fingers, close your eyes and visualize a favourite calming scene – a walk along a beach, perhaps, or sitting in a garden. Take a deep breath, and on the out breath pull downward and off very slowly. Have a drink of water and you will now feel ready to continue your work.

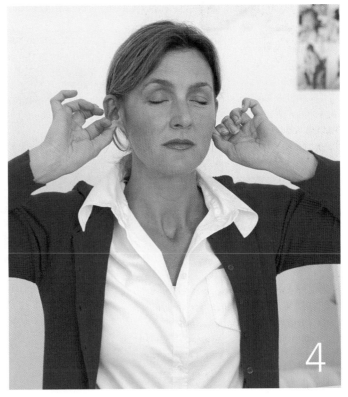

Seated Routine

If you have a reasonable amount of time to spare – during your lunch break, for instance – this seated routine through the clothes will allow you to work on a colleague's back as well as her neck and shoulders, which are the main areas of tension suffered by office and computer workers. Some large organizations employ a 'corporate' or 'on-site' massage therapist as part of their health programme, and a specially designed massage chair is used for the comfort of the receiver and accessibility for the giver. You can use an ordinary office chair, but not one with wheels.

1

Start by making your partner feel quite comfortable with your touch. Bring both hands down slowly and place them palm down on your partner's shoulders. Hold for 30 seconds, while your partner closes her eyes and relaxes in preparation for the massage.

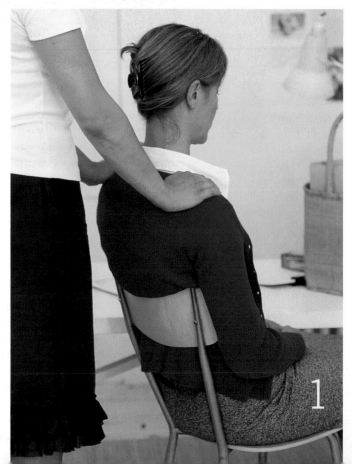

2

Working the area between the spine and the shoulder blades, use the heel of your hands and your fingers to lift and squeeze the muscle at the same time.

Repeat three to five times.

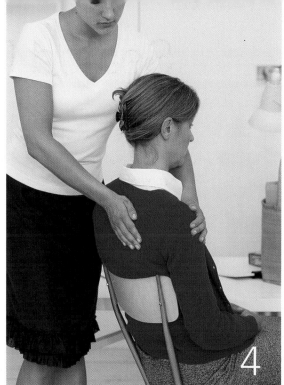

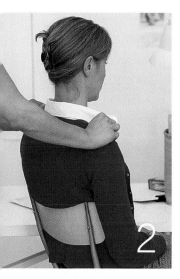

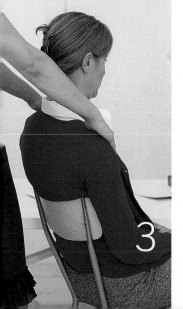

3

Placing your fingers over her shoulders, rotate the pads of your fingers across the muscle in the triangle between the collarbone and shoulders. Lean back slightly to apply pressure – the further you lean back, the stronger the pull, but always stick to a level that is acceptably comfortable for your partner.

Repeat three to five times.

4

Move side-on to your partner and place one arm across her upper chest area for support. Use the heel of your other hand to massage in circular movements over the back and shoulder area. Vary the speed from a gentle to a quite invigorating pace to warm up the muscles and increase the flow of both blood and lymph.

Repeat three to five times.

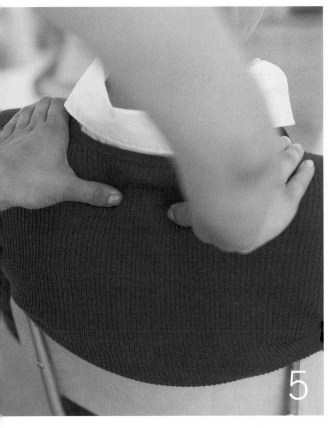

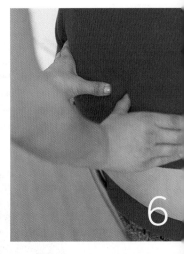

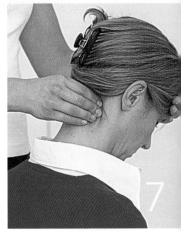

5

Now that the muscles are more relaxed, you can knead and apply deeper pressure. Stand behind your partner and, with your thumbs either side of the spine and using the pads only, apply on-the-spot pressure at 3cm (1¼in) intervals along the tops of the shoulder muscles, working outward and then returning.

6

Using the same technique as step 5, press your thumbs simultaneously on either side of the spine, working slowly down to the lower back area and then returning. If you want to reach the lower back, where most people experience discomfort, you can get your partner to straddle the chair.

7

Move to one side of your partner and support her forehead with the hand nearest to her. Ask her to rest her head on your hand and then place your free hand on the back of the neck area and squeeze the muscles between your fingers and thumb. Work upward to the base of the skull, then slide your fingers back to the starting position, ready to repeat.

8

Return to your position behind your partner and, standing straight, place the backs of your forearms on the top of her shoulders so that your palms are facing upward. Make sure your wrists are relaxed, take a deep breath, and on the out breath lean gently and slowly into the muscle, hold and then release. Work with your own breathing – keep the pressure on for the duration of your out breath and release it with your in breath.

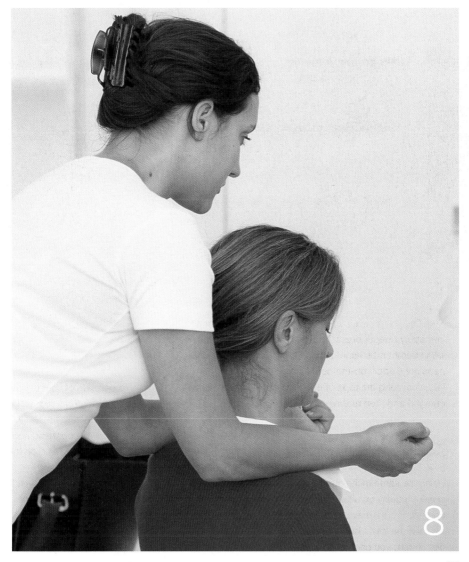

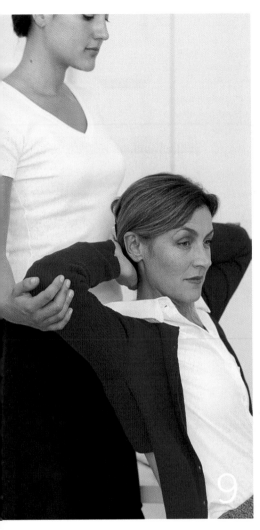

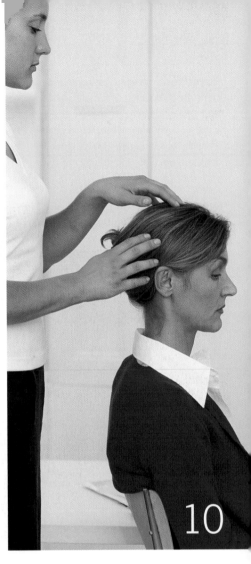

9

Ask your partner to clasp her hands behind her head, level with her ears. Hold her elbows firmly with your hands and ask her to take a deep breath. As she breathes out, slowly pull her arms straight back toward you to a comfortable point of resistance, hold for five seconds and then release. This will give an excellent stretch to the front chest and open up the respiratory area.

10

Start to bring the routine to a close. Rest your hands lightly on the crown of your partner's head and stroke from the forehead over to the base of the neck and down the back with a hand-over-hand motion.

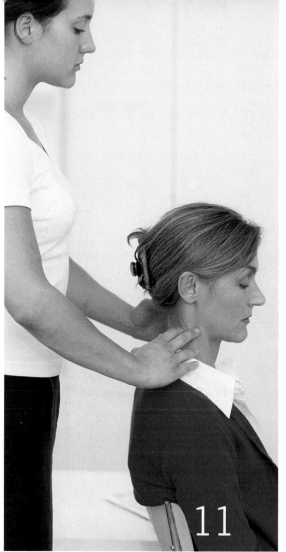

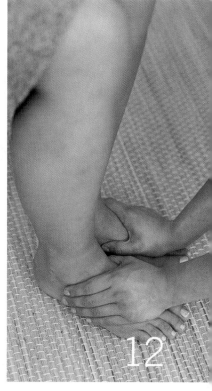

11

With both hands working simultaneously, move down the sides of your partner's head and tops of her shoulders in a gentle stroking movement, then squeeze down her arms to the elbows.

12

Finish off with a 'grounding' movement (see page 33) by holding your partner's feet with thumb pressure on the instep. Remember to offer her water before she returns to her desk.

Relaxing Massage

Just before going to bed is an ideal time to enjoy a deep, relaxing massage. Take a long, warm bath or shower beforehand to help relax the muscles that have been working hard all day. Tensions from long, stressful days in the office, overworked muscles or aches and stiffness from sitting at a desk all day rise to the surface and all can benefit from massage. At the same time, massage is a channel for communication with your partner and is as therapeutic to give as it is to receive. Enhance your massage with the use of oils to suit your mood and encourage a good night's sleep.

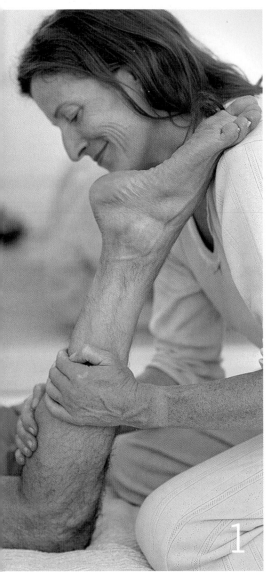

Lower Legs

This routine will promote relaxation of the calf, improve circulation and help to eliminate toxins from the body.

1

Position yourself at your partner's feet, then ask him to flex his knee and rest the top of his foot on your shoulder. Cup your hands either side of the calf muscles one above the other and use petrissage (see page 26) to apply even pressure, squeezing in opposite directions between your fingers and the heels of your hands, then release.

Repeat three to five times.

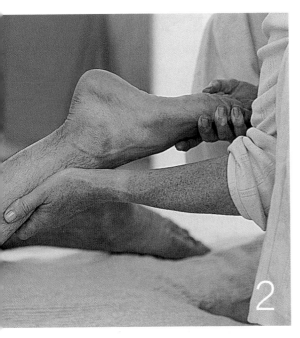

2

Gently take your partner's foot from your shoulder and hold it in one hand, supporting the underside of the leg with the other. Place your thumb in the groove on the outer edge of the leg and effleurage (see page 24) from above the ankle to the knee with pressure from your thumb and the flat of your hand. Take the pressure off while remaining in contact and glide back to the starting position.

Repeat three to five times.

3

Lower your partner's leg further, still supporting the ankle with one hand, and place your other hand palm down on the top of the calf. Effleurage from the ankle to the knee with pressure on the upward stroke, returning down the side of the leg.

Repeat three to five times.

Move to the other leg and repeat steps 1–3.

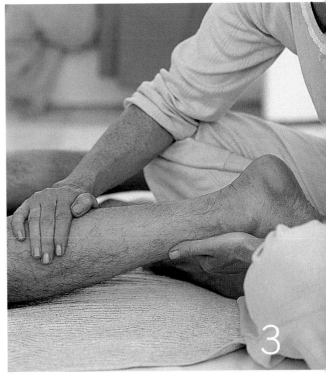

Back and Shoulders

These movements should release tension in the lower back area and help to mobilize the shoulders.

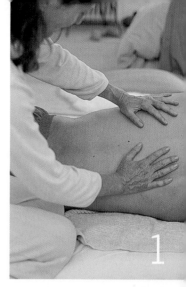

1

Position yourself to your partner's side at about hip level and ask him to lie comfortably on his side with his back toward you. Gently place the flats of both hands, one on either side of the spine, on the lower back area and effleurage (see page 24) up toward the shoulders, returning down the sides of the torso, with pressure on the upward stroke. This stroke is used to warm up the area and apply the oil.

Repeat three to five times.

2

Place one hand on your partner's shoulder to maintain contact, then make a fist with the other and, using knuckling (see page 30), lean in and work up the back along the side of the spine to the shoulder, returning down the side of the torso with the flat of your hand.

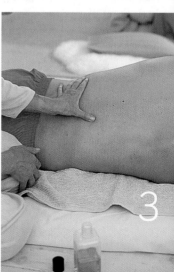

Repeat the stroke three to five times, then move to the other side of the spine and repeat the process.

3

Place the thumb and fingers of one hand either side of the spine, so that the web of your thumb straddles the vertebrae. Flex your thumb slightly and with the tip push up the back in 5cm (2in) long strokes until you have covered the whole area, gliding back with the flat of your hand to calm the area.

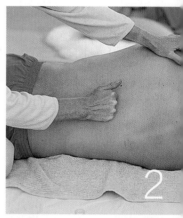

Repeat the movement three to five times before moving to the other side.

4

Place your thumbs either side of the
lower spine and effleurage up to the
shoulders, then return with flat hands
down the sides of the torso.

Repeat three to five times.

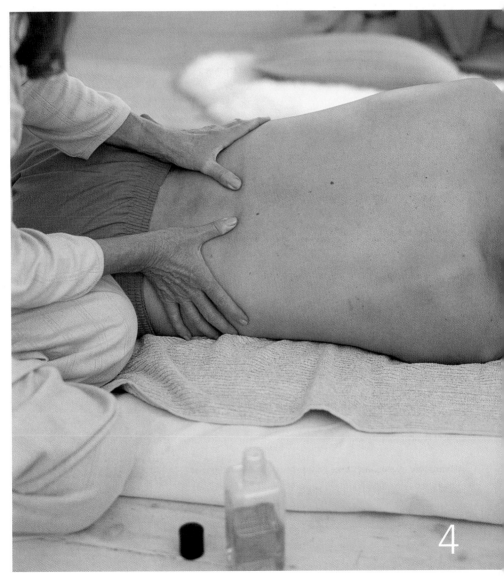

4

Neck and Shoulders

Neck stiffness and shoulder aches will respond to this sequence.

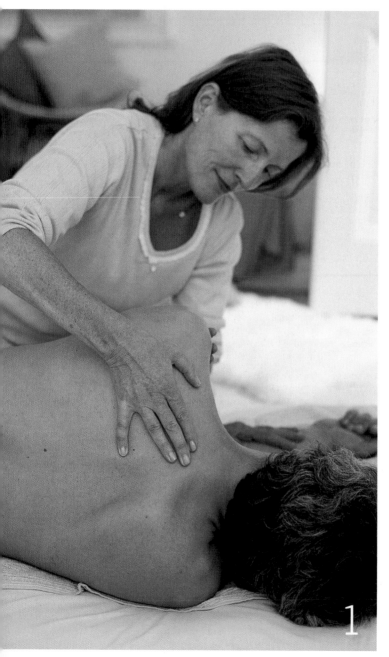

1

With your partner lying in the same position as for the back and shoulders sequence (see pages 66–7), move around to face him. Supporting the front of the shoulder with one hand, place the flat of the other on the shoulder blade and, with pressure on the upward stroke, effleurage (see page 24) up over the area toward the base of the neck.

Repeat three to five times.

2

Place your hands palm down, one on the front of the shoulder joint and the other on the back, sandwiching the shoulder and collarbone. Effleurage toward the neck, applying gentle pressure on the downward stroke and a slight pull on the return. This will stretch the neck and shoulder muscles.

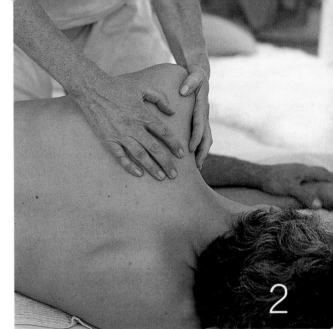

3

Once again working from behind, rest one hand on the top of the shoulder and make a fist with the fingers of the other hand. Place the flat of the fist, not the knuckles, at the base of the neck and, keeping flat to the surface, effleurage to the edge of the shoulder, then ease off the pressure, lift and return to the base of the neck. Adjust the pressure according to the response of your partner to avoid causing any discomfort.

Repeat several times.

Ask your partner to lie on his other side and repeat steps 1–3.

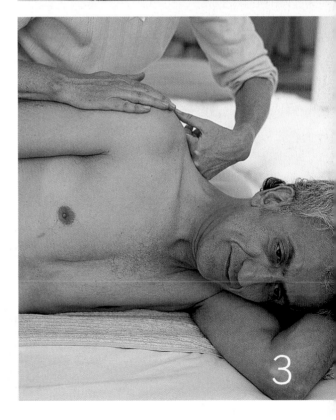

Knees

Legs and knees often suffer from fatigue and sometimes swell in the evenings, as they have been carrying the heavy weight of our bodies all day. The following movements will help to mobilize the knees.

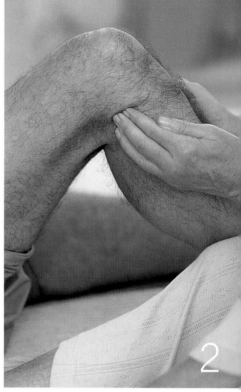

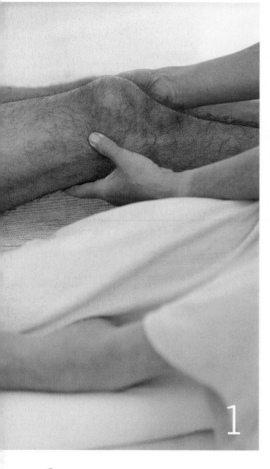

1

With your partner lying face up, position yourself to his side so that you can reach the knee area without overstretching. Place your hands on either side of the knee and gently effleurage (see page 24) around the area to ease and warm the joint.

2

Ask your partner to flex his knee and with one hand on either side of the joint, use your finger pads to effleurage in circular movements up and around the area. This will encourage blood flow around the knee, which in turn will ease tension and stiffness.

3

Supporting one side of the knee with one hand, place your other thumb just above the top of the joint. Using the pad, work upward in a curved line using short strokes, gradually covering the whole of the area. This will help to disperse any toxins or excess fluid.

Repeat steps 1–3 several times until the joint feels mobilized, then move to the opposite leg and repeat the process.

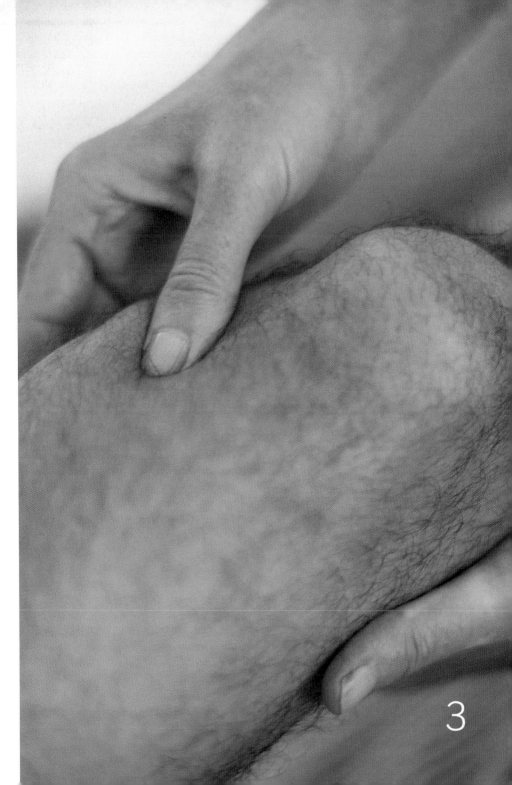

3

Thighs

The muscles in the thighs are usually overworked and need deeper work to break down the tensions and tightness.

1

With your partner lying face down, position yourself between the legs at knee level. Make a fist with both hands then knuckle (see page 30) hand over hand from the knee to the top of the thigh, lifting off at the end of the stroke and returning the hands to the knee.

Repeat the stroke three to five times.

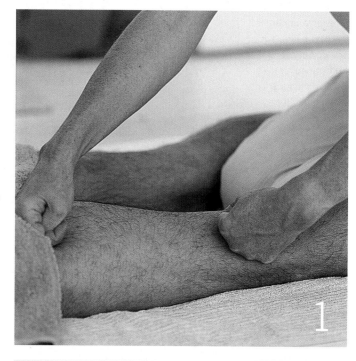

2

Place both hands flat down on the back of your partner's thigh, with one thumb on top of the other. Applying pressure with both thumbs, glide up the back of the thigh, returning with one hand on either side of the leg.

Repeat the stroke three to five times.

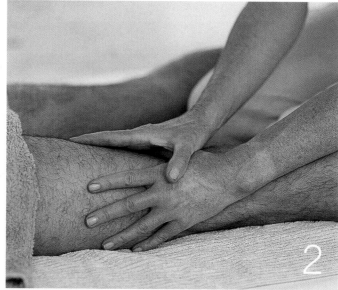

3

Move side-on to your partner, positioning yourself away from the leg on which you are working. Place both hands on the back of the thigh and wring the muscles (see page 27), leaning inward to apply firm pressure. Moving the hands in opposite directions and in a continuous rhythmic movement, work across the whole of the area.

Move to the other leg and repeat steps 1–3.

SAFETY FIRST

Be careful never to press hard when massaging the back of the knee as it is sensitive and it would be easy to cause pain.

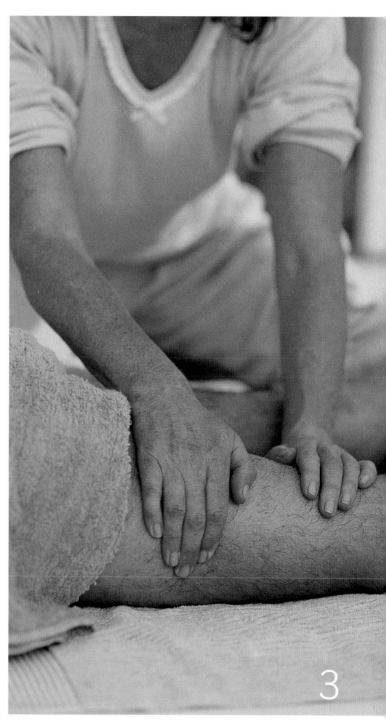

3

Feet

The soles of the feet contain thousands of nerve endings that connect to other parts of the body. Most people love having their feet massaged because it affects the whole of the body and makes them feel revitalized. The feet are very complex parts of our anatomy and act as the body's shock absorbers.

2

Supporting the heel and ankle firmly in one hand, wrap the fingers of the other hand around the top of the foot for extra support and to counterbalance the pressure. Massage using the thumb pad in a circling stroke, starting at the heel and ending just under the toes.

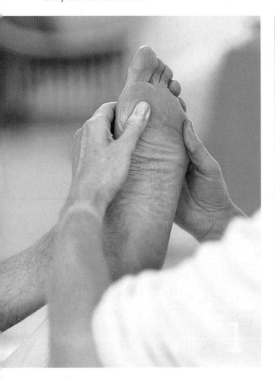

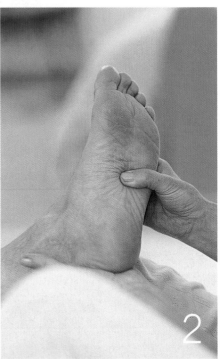

1

With yourself and your partner in a comfortable position, take one foot in both hands with the sole facing you. Wrap your fingers around the top of the foot and place one thumb on the ball. Using the whole length of your thumbs, apply pressure and pull the thumbs in opposite directions out toward the edge of the foot, lift off and return, ready to repeat. Work all across the length and width of the ball of the foot.

3

Place your hands on the top and sole of the foot and very gently effleurage (see page 24) down from the ankle and, leaning back slightly, pull off over the toes. This is a wonderful stroke with which to finish off and to make your partner feel the massage is complete.

Repeat several times.

Move to the other foot and repeat steps 1–3.

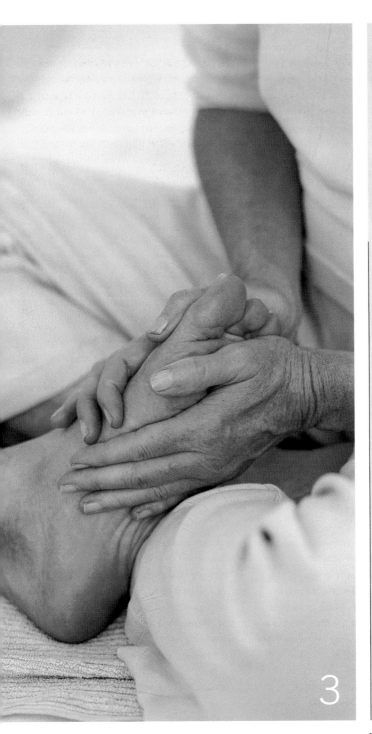

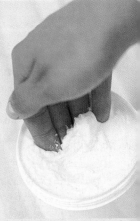

Tip

As an alternative to massage oil use a soothing peppermint foot lotion or a rich cream for a more luxurious feel. This will have the added benefit of moisturizing dry skin, which is common on this area of the body.

When you are massaging the feet, it is important that you apply a firm touch so that you do not tickle your partner.

3

Arms and Hands

Arm massage is great for releasing pent-up emotions. Use these strokes as an open channel of communication between yourself and your partner.

1

Take your partner's hand in yours, and with the flat of your other hand effleurage (see page 24) up the arm from the wrist to the shoulder, lessening the pressure slightly over the elbow joint. When you reach the top of the arm, glide over the shoulder and return down the underside of the arm to your starting position.

Repeat three to five times.

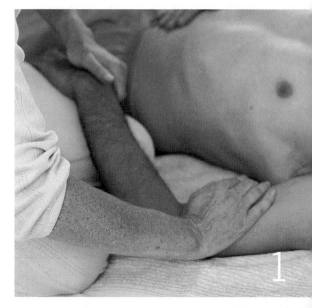

2

Still clasping the hand, place your other thumb across the inner wrist and squeeze up from the wrist to the elbow, rocking forward at the same time, then glide back with no pressure. You may find your partner's fingers opening and closing, as the muscles that control the fingers are located in the forearm.

Repeat three to five times.

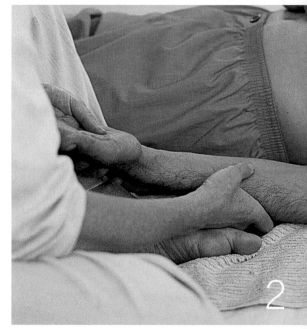

3

Move to the upper arm and, using petrissage (see page 26), squeeze the muscle between your fingers and the heel of your hand, working up its length and 'milking' all the tension out of the area.

Repeat three to five times, then smooth over with effleurage strokes.

Move to the other arm and repeat steps 1–3.

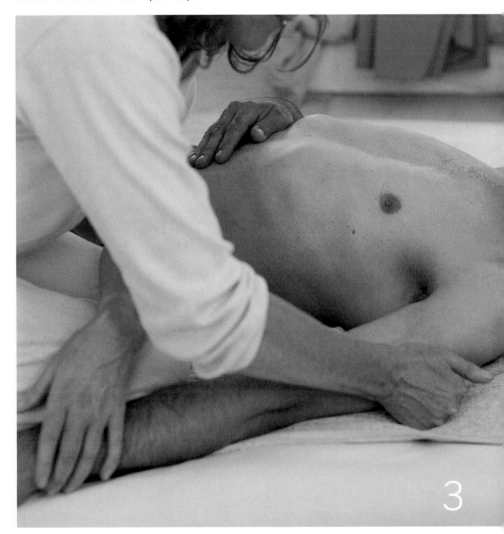

Face

Most massage to the face is based on shiatsu, which means 'finger pressure' in Japanese. Instead of long strokes, acupressure points are used to balance the body's energy. Gentle enough to relax, the pressure should feel firm but also caressing. We reflect tension and stress in our face with a tightening of the brow and jaw; calm and relaxation shows as a very 'open' face. Massaging the face enables us to drop some of our 'masks' and leads to a sense of deep relaxation.

SAFETY FIRST

Before you begin any face massage, you should make sure your partner is not wearing contact lenses.

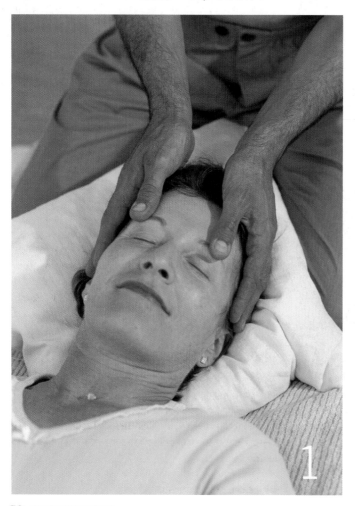

1

Make contact by resting the flats of your thumbs next to each other on the centre of your partner's forehead. Glide the flat of each thumb across the forehead to the outer edge, lift off and return, working on the whole area from the hairline to the brow.

2

Taking care, glide the thumbs across the eyebrows, working from the inner brow outward and off at the sides of the head. This movement soothes the whole of the eyebrow area.

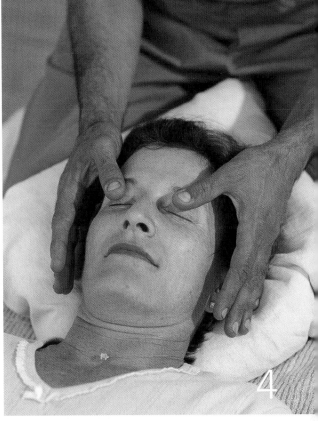

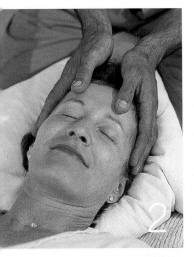

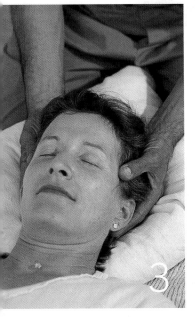

3

Place the pads of your thumbs on your partner's temples, resting in the natural hollow. With your fingers supporting the head behind the ears, make tiny circles over the temples. Alternatively, keep the thumbs stationary and press inward, hold for a few seconds and release. This is an excellent remedy for tension and headaches.

4

Ask your partner to close their eyes, if she has not already done so. Bringing your thumbs inward, start at the corner of the eye and carefully and lightly glide over the eyelids to the outer edge, then return. If the eyes are too sensitive, or your partner is too nervous, do the stroke but without making contact.

Repeat two or three times.

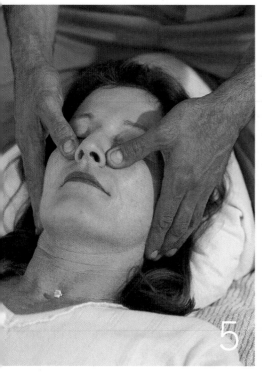

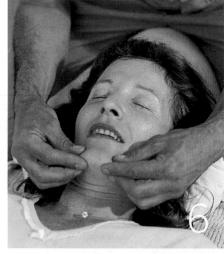

5

Starting from the top of the nostril, glide the tip of each thumb alongside the nose, sweep along the top of the cheekbone to the outer edge, pull off and return. This stroke follows the path of the sinuses and will help release any congestion (see also page 90).

Repeat once or twice.

6

Place your thumbs and fingers on the jawline, just either side of the centre and, in a rotatary movement, work each hand slowly outward toward the ears. You may notice that as the jaw relaxes your partner's mouth will open slightly, as a reflex to the massage and a sign that the tension held there is releasing.

7

When you reach the ears, pull down gently and off at the edges with your whole thumb. This is a very pleasurable stroke. Eastern philosophies believe that the ear is connected to – and represents – the whole of the body, so with this small movement your partner may feel relaxed all over.

8

Take the ears between your fingers and thumbs and gently pull outward, stretching them away from the head. Then squeeze all around the lobes, holding for a few seconds before breaking contact.

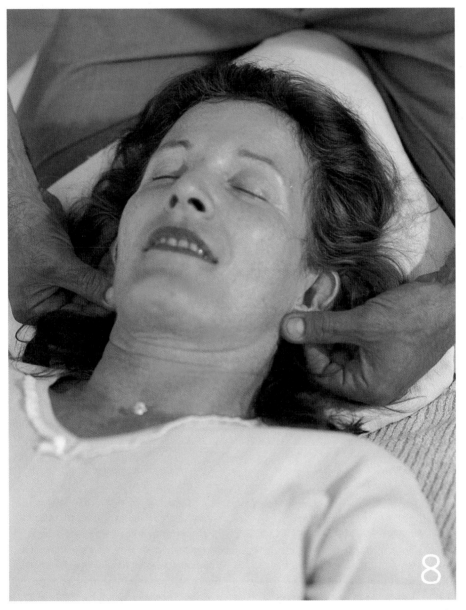

9

Move to the top of the head at hairline level and run your hands through your partner's hair, making sure that the tops of your fingers brush the whole of the scalp from front to back.

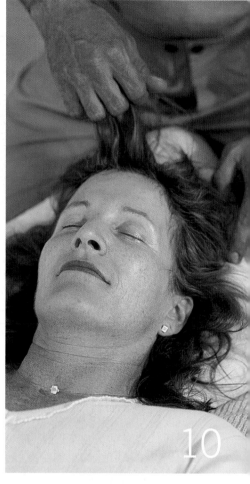

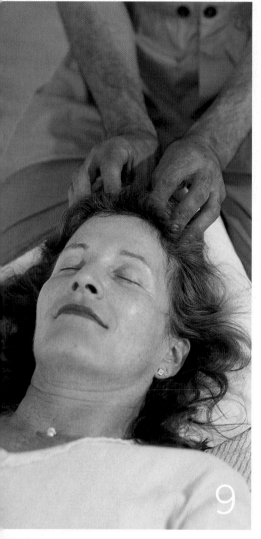

10

Take small strands of your partner's hair at a time and pull toward you very gently, working in sections over the whole of the head.

11

By now your partner should almost have drifted off and will be ready for bed. To finish, place the flat of one hand across the whole of the forehead with the other hand on top and hold for five to ten seconds.

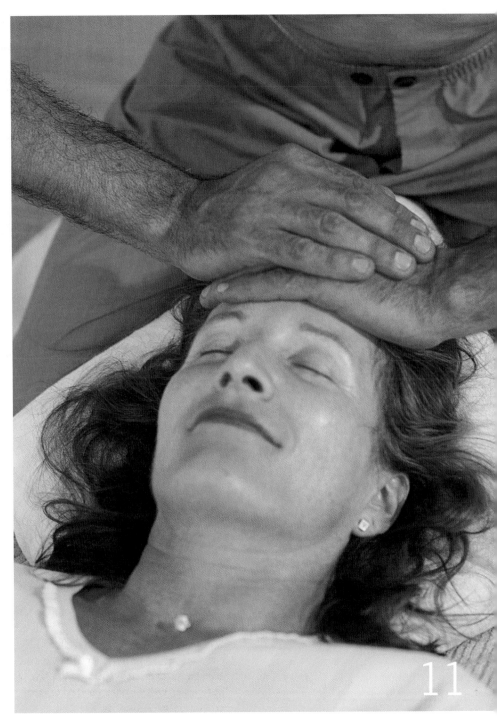

11

Head, Neck and Shoulders

Often the most relaxing part of a massage, work on the head, neck and shoulders deserves special attention as it is frequently here that we build up excessive tension. Take time with the strokes and give the massage with care.

1

Position yourself at your partner's head and make sure you are comfortable, as any slight movement will be transferred to your partner during this sequence. Turn your partner's head slightly away from the side you are massaging and with the other hand on the opposite shoulder for contact, start at the top of the neck and glide your hand downward using effleurage (see page 24) to the edge of the shoulder. Turn your hand slightly to return, scooping up the neck with the web of your hand.

Repeat three to five times, then move to the other side of the neck and repeat.

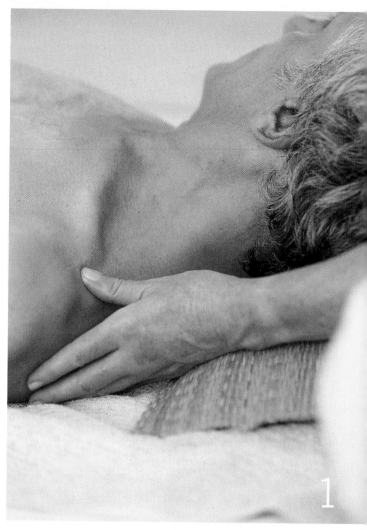

1

2

Cupping your hands over your partner's ears with your fingers wrapped underneath, use the heels of your hands to pull slowly downward over the ears and off. Make sure the stretch is not so strong as to become uncomfortable.

Repeat several times.

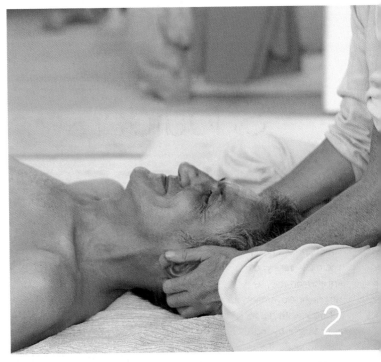

3

In order to turn your partner's head in a safe and confident way, hold it on either side with your thumbs above the ears and your fingers behind in a V shape, lift the head slightly and rest it on one hand that is cupped slightly. Do not pull on the hair and make sure that your partner feels comfortable, as, in order for the muscles to relax, you want him to relax into your hands and not resist.

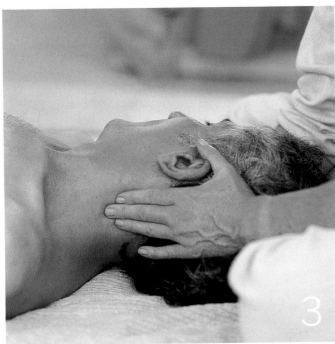

4

With your partner's head turned slightly away from the side being massaged, position the pads of your fingers along the base of his skull, press upward and slowly rotate your fingers in very tiny circles. Work along the area, cradling the rest of his head in your hands for support.

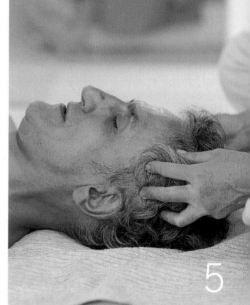

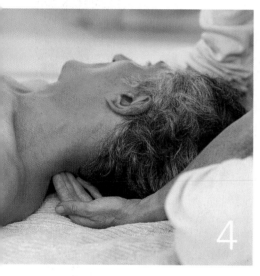

5

Using your fingers on either side of the head, press into the scalp and, in a 'shampooing' motion, work thoroughly over the whole head in a continuous, rhythmic movement. If you find this position difficult, use one hand only, remembering to keep contact with the other.

6

Move to a side position facing your partner, place your hands firmly over the tops of the shoulders and pull firmly toward you with the flats of your fingers. This is a gentle shoulder pull and should not raise the torso off the massage surface.

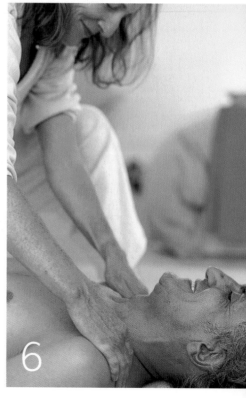

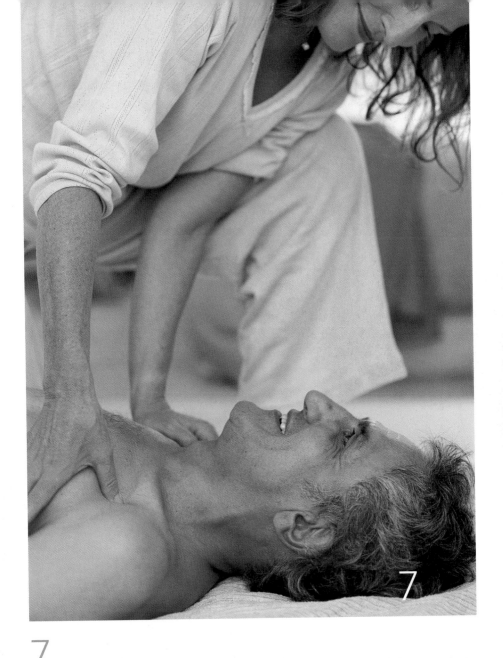

7

To release and relax this area further, with one hand resting on a shoulder place the other on the pectoral muscle (see page 16) at the front of the chest. With your thumb and the web of your hand, glide across the muscle to the outer edge.

Repeat two or three times, then move to the other side and repeat.

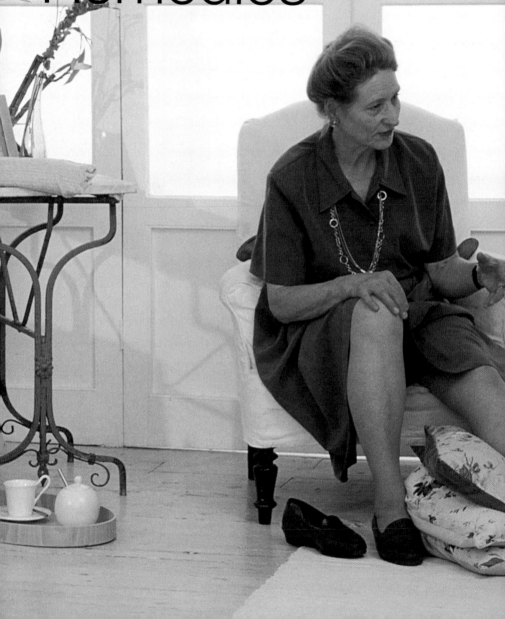

Massage
Remedies

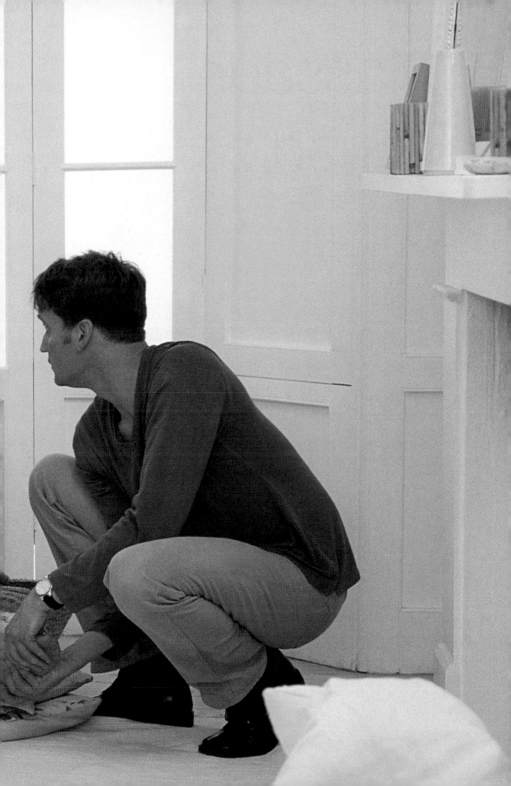

Sinusitis and Headaches

The most common complaints of the face and head area often respond very well to massage. The pain usually manifests itself at the base of the skull, the temples and forehead and at the top of the head, and is often caused by stress or bad posture. Migraine sufferers can also experience some relief, provided they feel comfortable enough to receive massage.

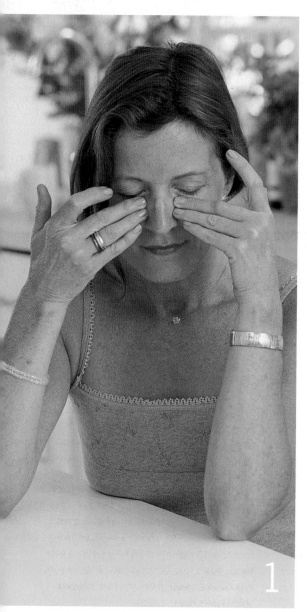

1 Sinusitis

The sinuses are hollow, air-filled cavities that drain into the nasal cavities. Congestion or inflammation of the sinuses results in a heavy, blocked-up feeling and pain in the face and head. Infection can be caused by such things as pollution or dirty water taken in while swimming. Self-massage is very effective because you can regulate the pressure according to the severity of the condition. Place your middle fingers on the sides of your nose, breathe in, and on the out breath glide your fingers down the sides of your nose to the nostrils and on to the cheeks, following the natural curve. Palpating the areas at the beginning and end of this sequence will also help to drain the sinuses.

Repeat several times.

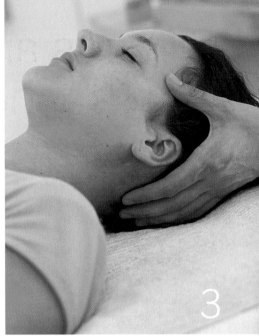

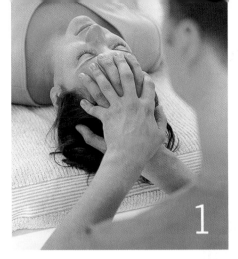

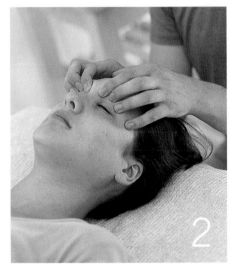

1 Headache

Slowly place one hand with your fingers spread on your partner's head and forehead. Placing your other hand on top, slowly lean your weight into your hands until a comfortable pressure is achieved, hold for about 15 seconds and then release without losing contact. This is a very subtle movement, but a headache in the forehead region can be relieved by this deep pressure.

Repeat four to five times.

2

Place the pads of your fingers just along the underside of the brow bones. Taking care not to apply too much pressure, because this area of the face can be quite tender, hold for about 15 seconds and then release without losing contact with your partner.

Repeat four to five times.

3

Move your hands to the sides of the head, with your thumbs positioned on the temples. Check with your partner that the pressure is comfortable and then slowly rotate the pads of your thumbs clockwise about 15 times – the slower the rotation, the more relaxing it will feel – then hold the pressure without rotating for about 15 seconds. Finish by bringing your hands down to cover both ears, wrapping your fingers underneath them and then drawing your fingers down and off.

Digestive Problems

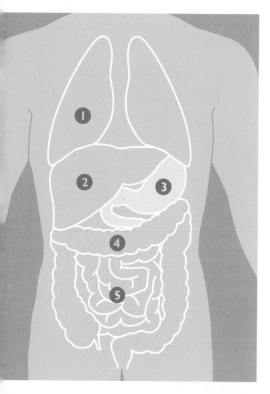

Our digestive processes tend to reflect our state of mind. Stress can cause all sorts of conditions in this area, including irritable bowel syndrome (see pages 94–5), ulcers, indigestion, constipation and diarrhoea. This is because the blood supply is inhibited, and this, in turn, affects the way the digestive system absorbs and distributes nutrients. In addition, the muscle wall of the intestinal tract, which pushes the food through the body by contracting, cannot function properly.

The abdomen is the most exposed and unprotected area of the body. In the East the *hara* (abdomen) is considered to house the body's vital energy. When massaging this area, be aware that your partner may feel vulnerable, so take some time to observe their breathing pattern and try to coordinate your strokes with this. Even the lightest touch may cause her to contract her abdominal muscles instinctively, so place your hands down gently. Before you start, pause for about 20 seconds to reassure your partner, lift off to apply oil and return gently, ready to start massaging.

DIGESTIVE SYSTEM

❶ lungs
❷ liver
❸ stomach
❹ large intestine
❺ small intestine

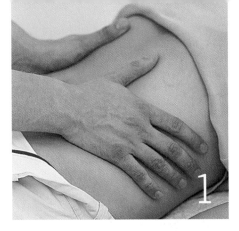

1

Using effleurage (see page 24), glide upward to just under the breast area and then, with your hands on either side of the torso, slowly return to your starting position. This stroke will calm and soothe the area and is particularly beneficial in relieving both abdominal bloating and indigestion.

Repeat five times in a flowing movement.

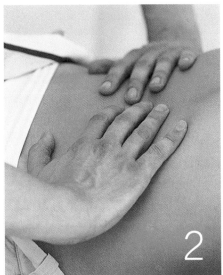

2

Always apply this stroke after you have relaxed the area with step 1. Using the flat of your hands and gentle pressure, on your partner's out breath draw your hands apart diagonally (left ribs to right hip, for example), working outward in a sweeping action and remembering that this is more of a stretching movement than working deeply. This will help to release contracted muscle and so is excellent for menstrual cramping. Using a massage oil blended with chamomile, lavender or rose can provide additional relief.

Repeat in the other direction.

3

Place one hand on top of the other and, making sure that your whole hand is in contact with your partner, work in a circular, clockwise movement from the solar plexus following the direction of the large intestine (see diagram, opposite). Start with a large circle and continue, reducing the size of the circle but increasing the pressure, for a further four or five times. Remember to follow your partner's breathing with your hands. You will find this movement helpful for relieving abdominal pain and constipation.

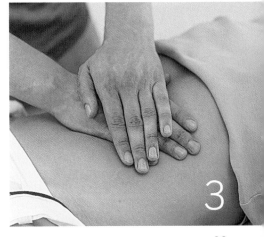

Irritable Bowel Syndrome (IBS)

This is a collective term for disorders of the bowel. Massage can be very effective in relaxing the area and so reducing spasm of the involuntary muscles.

1

After warming up the area with gentle effleurage (see page 24), position yourself side-on to your partner and place your hands on opposite sides of the abdomen, cupped slightly over the sides of the torso. Using equal pressure and even weight on your palms and fingers, push one hand forward and the other back in a petrissage motion (see page 26), covering the whole of the abdomen from near side to far side.

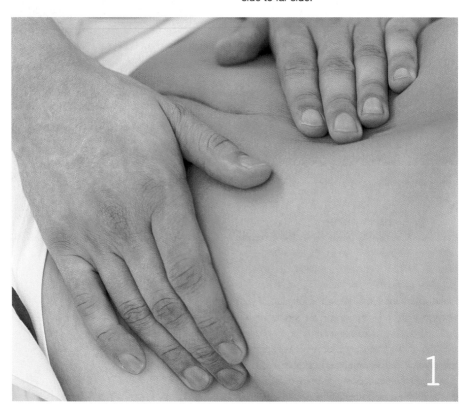

1

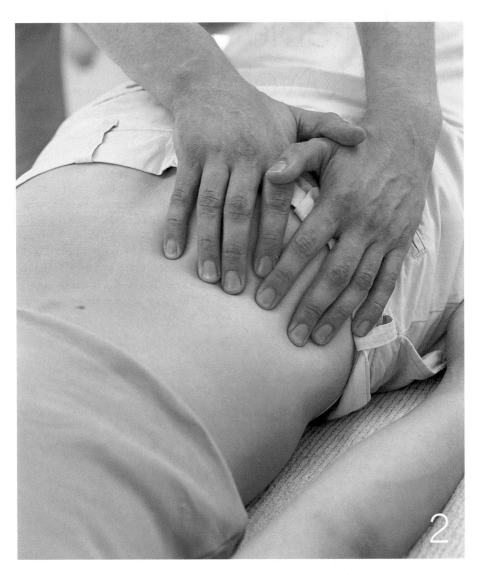

2

Place your hands just below the left side of your partner's ribcage, with your fingers spread and facing up toward her head. This is a vibrational technique: as you apply pressure with the pads of your fingers, make very small circular movements with each fingertip simultaneously. This massages the descending colon and helps to move its contents more smoothly along the digestive tract.

Asthma

Characterized by intermittent wheezing and breathlessness, asthma is one of several common symptoms of respiratory stress. This distressing condition is much more common now. The difficulty in breathing is caused by spasm and inflammation of the bronchial tubes and their mucus lining, and by a tightening of the chest muscle.

The frequency and severity of attacks are often related to emotional states such as stress and anxiety. This is where massage can play a very beneficial role, even being applied during an attack in a sitting position if the sufferer is comfortable with this. Remember to relax and warm up the area with gentle effleurage (see page 24) before applying the following specific movements.

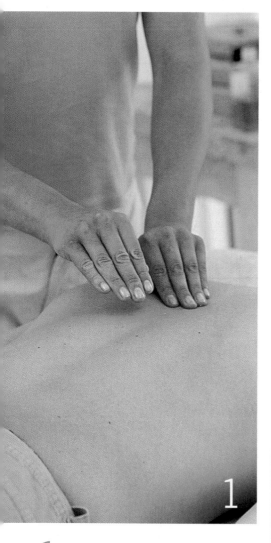

1

SAFETY FIRST

Used on a regular basis, massage will help the asthma sufferer to maintain a relaxed state and may contribute toward alleviating the condition. However, there are times when massage would not be appropriate:

• When there is a respiratory tract infection
• During an unrelenting attack
• If medication has not had any effect

Massage is *not* a substitute for medication and any changes in medication arising from the benefits of massage should be discussed with your doctor first.

1

Cup (see page 29) over the back area, avoiding the spine. Usually this movement is administered between attacks, when the sufferer is more comfortable, and helps to release any build-up of mucus.

2

Flick (see page 29) to apply friction to the spaces between the ribs (intercostals). This will stimulate the local circulation, help to promote lymph flow and relax the muscles in this area.

3

Passive movements help the expansion of the whole area, which is very useful if the sufferer is unable to exercise. Standing upright at your partner's head, place his hands around your lower back. Support his upper arms just above the elbows, and ask him to take a deep breath. As he inhales, flex your knees and lean backward. Maintain this stretch while he exhales and then ease off, keeping hold of his arms, and straighten your knees.

Repeat once.

4

For a bigger stretch, slide your hands down to your partner's forearms with his hands gripping yours and repeat step 3, stretching on his in breath and holding as he breathes out.

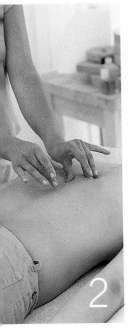

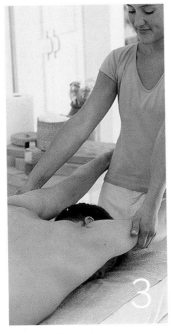

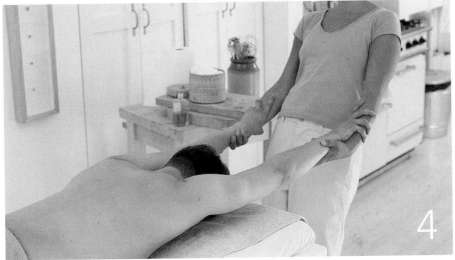

Menstruation and Menopause

Every month many women suffer from one or many of the effects of their hormonal cycle – water retention, headaches, pelvic congestion resulting in back ache, cramping and pain – caused by hormone imbalance. By inducing relaxation, massage can reduce the symptoms of premenstrual tension, such as irritability, depression and crying spells. It can also release tightness in muscles and stimulate the blood and lymph flows, thereby helping in the elimination of toxins and excess fluid. It is, however, very important to work within the sufferer's comfort level, as sometimes she may feel too tense and sensitive for anything other than very light strokes.

During the menopause, a different kind of hormonal imbalance causes symptoms that include sweating, hot flushes, migraines and bloating. There are trigger points within the abdominal wall that, when treated, can bring relief – this is in contrast to abdominal massage, which can sometimes increase blood pressure and produce hot flushes. Gentle massage is ideal for reducing the musculoskeletal pain that is sometimes a characteristic of menopause.

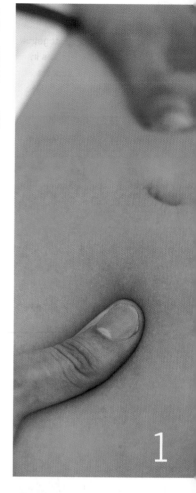

1

Place the pads of your thumbs about 7cm (3in) on either side of your partner's navel and, using your body weight, lean in toward the navel and hold for five seconds.

Repeat two or three times.

2

Move your thumbs close together and, using the pads, work as in step 1 downward in a straight line, from just below the navel to end level with the hips, then work back up, finishing with your thumbs about 7cm (3in) to either side of your partner's navel. This will relax stomach tension and reduce spasms and fatigue.

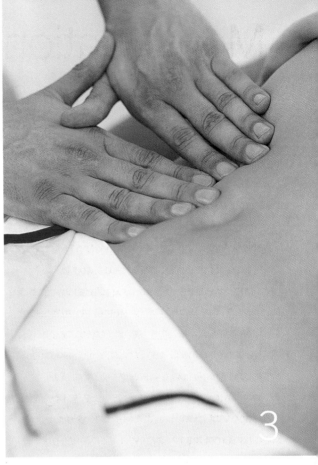

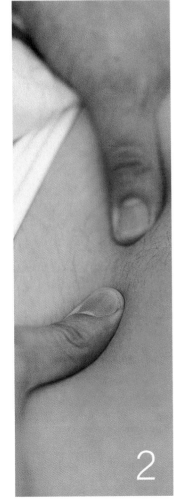

3

Relax your hands by shaking them and place them lightly, close together, on the mid-abdomen, level with the navel, and effleurage (see page 24) lightly and gently in an arc toward the groin and return. Make sure that you massage both sides of the abdomen equally. As you become more experienced, you may wish to use an intermittent pressure technique instead of the gliding stroke. To do this, use mostly the pads of your fingers and, instead of sliding, 'stretch' the tissues by alternately applying pressure and releasing as you move in an arc toward the groin. This is a very subtle movement and you should keep contact with your partner at all times. The technique works on the lymphatic flow and is especially effective in reducing water retention in the abdominal area.

Oedema

Derived from the Greek word meaning 'to swell', an oedema is simply an excess of fluid inside or between cells. It can be situated in one specific area or may spread throughout the body. There are many causes, from minor problems, such as premenstrual water retention and 'housemaid's knee' caused by too much kneeling or the effects of a hot climate, to more serious problems, including heart or kidney failure and lymphoedema (swollen lymph nodes). Massage can be effective in dealing with some of the simpler problems, but treatment for more complex conditions requires professional training and, in some cases, a doctor's approval. The techniques shown here can also be adapted for self-massage.

1

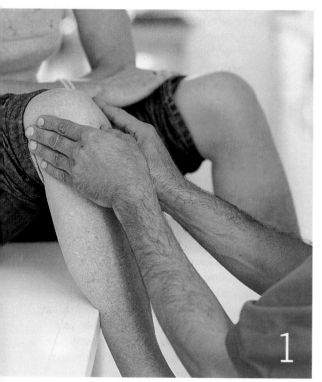

This technique is useful for dispelling 'water on the knee'. Using the pads of your thumbs, work around the knee joint, starting at the top. Lean into the area surrounding the kneecap and move downward on each side, applying pressure slowly and to a level that is comfortable for your partner. Direct the pressure inward toward the centre and hold for five seconds before moving to the next position, until you have reached the area under the joint, completing the circle.

Repeat on the other leg.

To finish off, move to the feet and hold for 20 seconds to 'ground' your partner (see page 33).

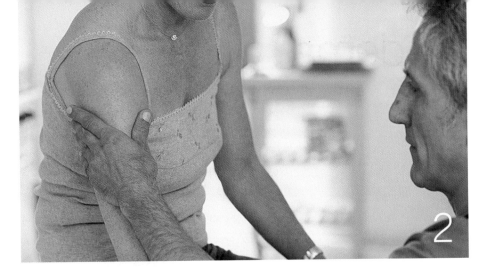

2

A build-up of fluid in the upper arm can result from over-exercising, hormonal changes during menstruation, poor lymph flow or from removal of the lymph nodes during a mastectomy. Support your partner's arm by holding the inside of their elbow and rest their forearm on yours. Using your other hand, lean into the outside of the upper arm and with your fingers and thumb squeeze over the muscle, slowly working upward from the elbow to the shoulder. Return with flat-handed effleurage (see page 24) down the outside of the arm. This movement is great for improving the circulation.

Repeat up to five times before moving to the other arm.

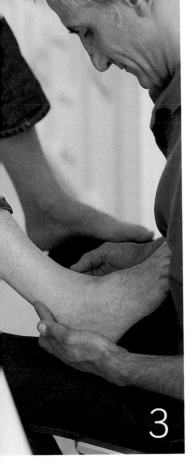

3

One of the most obvious areas of fluid build-up is around the feet and ankles. Long periods of walking on hot summer days, aeroplane cabin pressure or tight footwear will all result in a 'puffy' look, which can be eased by a simple 'drainage' massage. Supporting the foot, make small circular movements with your fingers, always working around and not directly on the swelling. Then, with your fingers under the heel for support, press your thumb pads simultaneously on both sides of the Achilles tendon and hold the pressure for five seconds.

Travel Problems

However we travel, and whether we are young or old, from time to time most of us suffer from travel sickness. More recently a condition called deep vein thrombosis (DVT) has been identified. It is linked with sitting inactively for long periods of time as in an aeroplane or car and involves the formation of a blood clot, usually in the calf area, which causes swelling and pain. A more serious consequence arises if this clot then travels around the body and ends up lodged in the lung. Massage can help, as it helps the blood flow through the deep veins and their valves in the legs onward toward the heart, which would normally be achieved through movement and pressure.

TRAVEL REMEDIES

If you have to take a long trip, you can reduce the risk of DVT with a simple self-help programme.

- Keep your body hydrated by drinking plenty of water.
- Do not cross your legs, as this puts pressure on the blood vessels at the back of the legs.
- Make sure your socks and shoes are not constricting.
- Exercise your legs or, if possible, move about at regular intervals.
- If you suffer from varicose veins, clotting or have had a recent injury or surgery on your legs, consider wearing support hose or 'airline socks'.
- At intervals, apply some simple self-massage techniques.

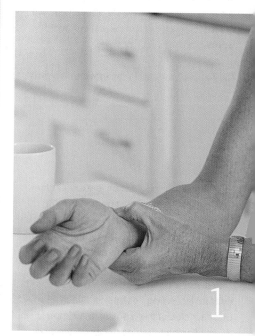

1 Motion Sickness

Massaging a particular pressure point on your wrist works in a similar way to the special wrist bands you can purchase at most pharmacies and can relieve sickness. Place the pad of your thumb on the inside of your other wrist in alignment with your first finger and apply pressure, using your fingers to support the back of the hand on which you are working.

Repeat on the other hand.

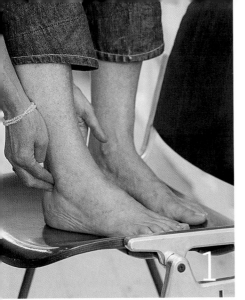

Deep Vein Thrombosis (DVT)

1

This is a simple technique, which you can apply while you are sitting. With both hands working on one leg, place the pads of your fingers on either side of your foot between the ankle and the heel. Working in small circular movements, apply intermittent pressure as though you are manually pumping the area.

Repeat on the other leg.

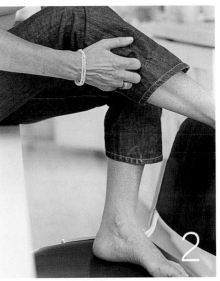
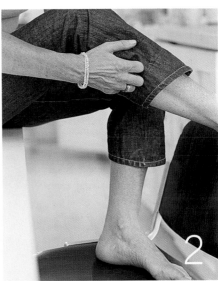

2

Knuckle (see page 30) both hands upward from the ankle toward the knee area and return, with the pressure always on the upward stroke. You can apply this pressure either in a straight or circular movement over the sides or back of the calves, but avoid working on any varicose veins.

Repeat five times and then move to work on the other leg.

3

This simple pumping action is excellent for maintaining good blood flow. In a rocking movement and using both feet simultaneously, lift your heels and then tap your toes. You can move your feet in the same or alternate directions – you may enjoy doing this to music. For a variation on this exercise, use an inflatable travelling neck pillow: place your feet on either side of the U shape and simply press down alternately, letting the air do the work.

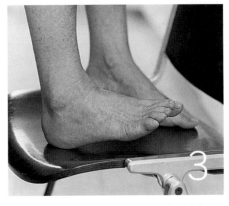

Tired Feet

If you have a job that requires a great deal of standing or walking, there is nothing as revitalizing as a foot massage – it is also a great way to end a hard day's shopping! It is a good massage to teach youngsters to do on each other, on parents and on grandparents. The routine can be used on its own or as a continuation of a leg massage. In addition to revitalizing tired feet, this sequence will relax tension caused by high arches and even prevent winter chilblains, which are caused by poor circulation.

1

Place the flat of your hands on the top of your partner's foot with one thumb on top of the other, ready to administer effleurage (see page 24). Using powder to help the glide, and light pressure, on your out breath work up the front of the foot toward the lower leg. When you reach this point, glide back down on either side of the foot, leaning back to add a slight pull to the stroke.

Repeat three to five times.

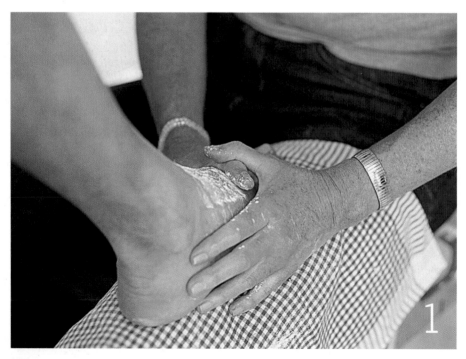

2

From a position that enables you to keep your arms straight, rest your thumbs and the heel of your hands on the top of the foot, with your fingers wrapped around the sides. Draw your thumbs across the foot in opposite directions, squeezing the foot firmly, and bring them down to join the rest of your hand in a movement that stretches and opens up the area.

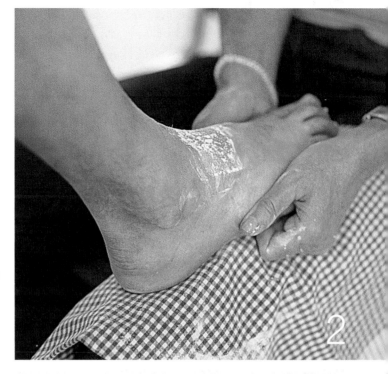

3

Make your hands into fists then knuckle (see page 30) all over the top and sides of the foot with circling movements.

Repeat this several times. Now use the same strokes on the other foot.

At the end of the routine, hold your partner's feet for 20 seconds in order to 'ground' her.

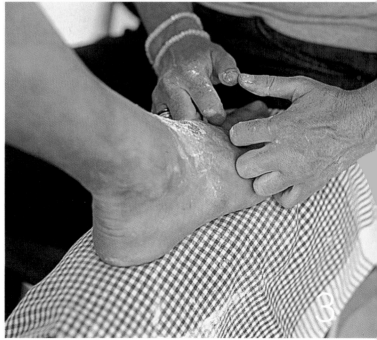

Calf Cramps

Calf cramps are muscle contractions that send the calf into spasm, and they may occur for no obvious reason. They can be alleviated with a simple kneading stroke (see page 27), which can also be adapted for self-massage.

1

With your fingers closed together, cup both hands around the back of your partner's calf so that the tips of the fingers of each hand are facing each other along the midline of the calf muscle. Exert pressure with both hands simultaneously and roll the muscle using the kneading stroke (see page 27), then release the pressure and repeat, slowly moving your hands up the whole length of the calf in order to reduce the muscle tension in it and relieve the spasm.

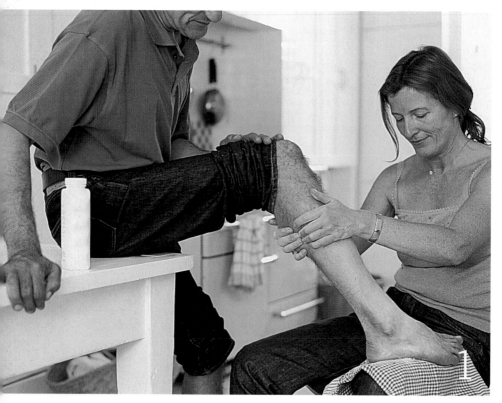

2

Supporting the ankle with one hand, flex the foot to its point of resistance by pushing the toes and ball of the foot forward with the other hand. Reverse the action by pulling back the foot with one hand while pushing down on the heel with the other. This will release and stretch the calf muscle and also increase blood flow to the area, slowly reducing the cramping.

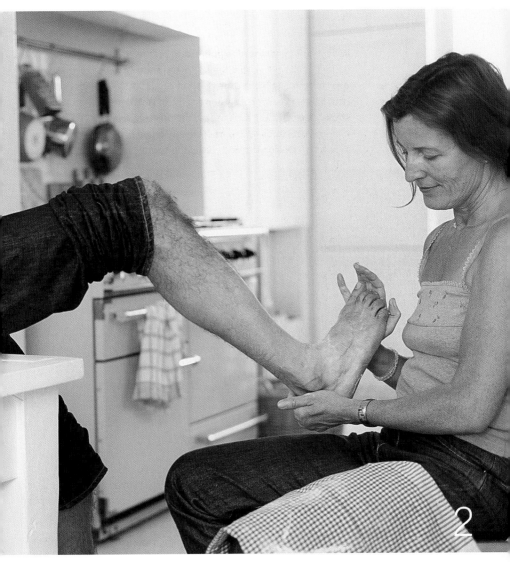

Eye Strain

In today's world of computer screens, electronic media and bright lights, eye strain is common and can cause blurred vision, headaches and even migraines. To counteract this, you can do this simple routine while sitting at a table or desk. Make sure you are sitting comfortably with your elbows on a firm surface so that you can hold the weight of your head in your hands. Oil is not necessary, although a small amount of rose absolute would add a special dimension to the massage.

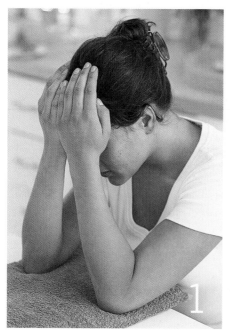

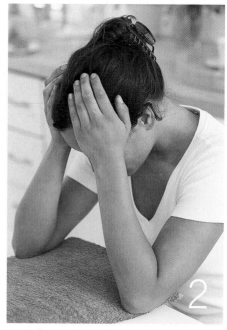

1

Place your fingers on the top of your head, rest your eyes into the heels of your hands and relax your whole body, letting your hands take the weight. Hold this position for 20 seconds and release.

Repeat four times.

2

Move the heels of your hands to rest on your eyebrows. Take a deep breath, and on the out breath glide your hands from the inner ends of your eyebrows outward and pull off at the side of the head, smoothing the entire browline.

Repeat four times.

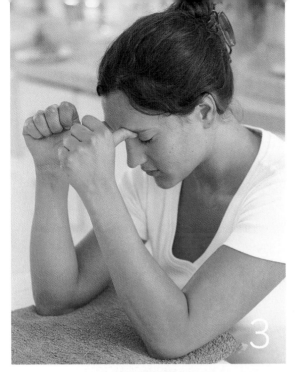

3

Place the pads of your thumbs underneath the inner edge of your eyebrows. As this is a very tender area, do not lean in with the whole weight of your head but stick to a level of pressure with which you are comfortable. Hold for ten seconds and release. This technique is not only good for tired eyes but also helps to clear congestion of the sinuses and related headaches (see pages 90–91).

Repeat four times.

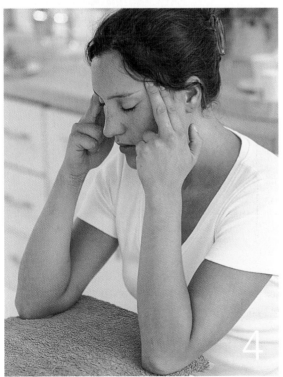

4

Finally, place the first and second fingers of each hand on your temples and, using the pressure from your fingers as support, release your head and neck. Take a deep breath, and on the out breath very slowly rotate your fingers clockwise. You can also apply the pressure directly to your temples without rotating your fingers.

Repeat the movement four times.

Insomnia and Anxiety

Insomnia is a side-effect of stress and is usually linked with anxiety about something in our lives. Massage promotes sleep naturally, which is very important in breaking the cycle of fatigue. The ideal time to massage is just before going to bed, and an essential oil such as lavender can be used to enhance the benefits of the massage. Use gentle, rhythmic strokes or a facial routine as shown here, and encourage your partner to let go of the thoughts of the day, empty their mind and drift.

1

Making sure your partner is nicely comfortable and warm, position yourself at her head and, leaning forward, place the fingers of both hands on her chin. With your finger pads rotating in small circles, move along around the jawline to just in front of the ear lobe. This is a very slow movement to expel the tension that is so often stored in this part of the face.

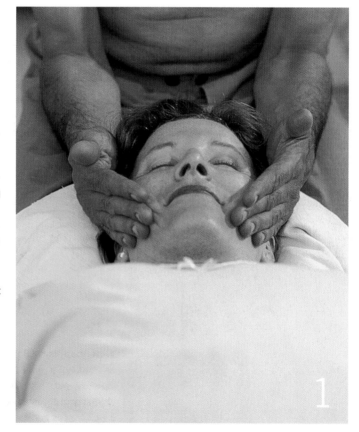

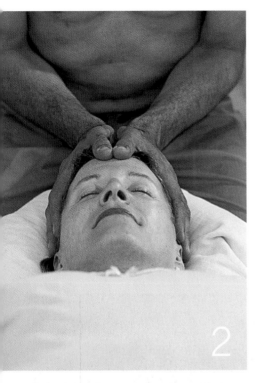

2

Place your thumbs together and flat to the surface at the centre of the forehead, holding the sides of the head. Glide each thumb outward to the temples, lift off and return to the centre of the forehead.

Repeat several times, moving up over the whole of the forehead to the hairline.

3

Place your thumbs one on top of the other at the centre of the forehead near the hairline, then exert pressure, hold for a few seconds and then release.

Repeat, moving up over the head.

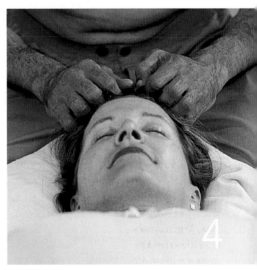

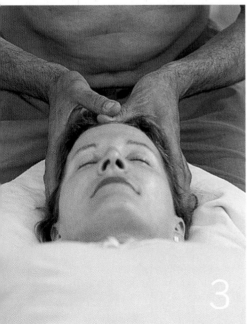

4

Draw the splayed fingers of both hands very slowly through your partner's hair in a combing action, moving one hand and then the other in a continuous, rhythmic motion. Be careful not to pull the hair sharply.

Repetitive Strain Injury (RSI)

RSI is finally being recognized as a real health problem relating to the workplace – but what exactly is it? It is actually a collective term used for carpel tunnel syndrome, non-specific arm pain, occupational overuse and work-related disorders of the arm. Although we often associate it with the strain of using a keyboard, it can be caused by any repetitive action, and it affects musicians, checkout operators and assembly-line workers alike. Even housework or a hobby involving a specific physical movement can be a cause. The simple routine shown here can be done at any time and anywhere. A good time is after work, perhaps while you and your partner are catching up on the day's events.

CHECK YOUR SYMPTOMS

The following are all symptoms of RSI:

- Weakness or loss of function in the muscles and joints of the hands, arms, shoulders or neck.
- Tingling, numbness or cold feelings in the hands and fingers.
- Swelling or a sense of swelling.
- Persistent pain even after resting.

HOW TO PREVENT RSI

Follow these guidelines to help you avoid RSI:
- Take regular breaks to avoid long periods of continuous, repetitive movement.
- Make sure your work station is ergonomically designed and sound.
- Concentrate on your posture. For desk work, make sure your wrists are kept straight and your forearms are supported.
- Practise stretching exercises for the hands, neck and shoulders at regular intervals.

If you think you have symptoms of RSI, do not ignore them or camouflage them with painkillers, as only body maintenance will bring relief. Acupuncture, the Alexander Technique for posture, and massage can all play a part in the prevention of RSI.

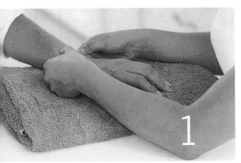

1

Using the pads of your thumbs and rotating them alternately in opposite directions, work in between and over the bony area of your partner's wrist.

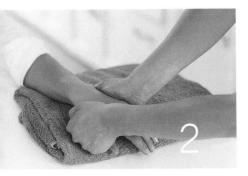

2

Starting with the heels of your hands on the centre back of your partner's hand, and your fingers wrapped around it, apply pressure and glide your hands in opposite directions across to the edge. This will really stretch and open up the whole area.

Repeat this step three to five times.

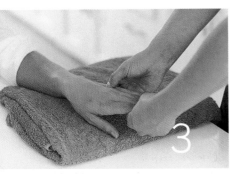

3

Place your thumb pad just above the web between your partner's third and fourth fingers, then apply pressure and glide up toward the wrist, following the hollow channel between the knuckles. Move to the web between the second and third fingers and repeat the movement, continuing in this way until you have worked your way right across the hand.

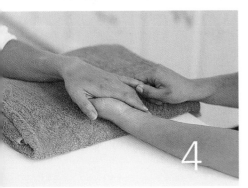

4

Supporting your partner's hand in a flat clasp, take the base of her little finger between your thumb and first finger and gently slide down, stretching and twisting as you go and pulling off at the tip. Move along the hand, working each finger and the thumb in the same way.

Move to the other hand and repeat steps 1–4.

Strained Knee

1

Strains and sprains are common injuries during sport and exercise and involve a tear in the muscle, usually caused by overdoing exercise, over-stretching or a bad movement. Massage helps by reducing the swelling that is a visible symptom of this type of injury – always work above the swelling and if the skin reddens, work higher. Reducing the swelling will automatically reduce the pain as well; however, if the area feels too sensitive to receive massage, you could palpate pressure points to achieve the same results (see page 17).

Place your hands on either side of your knee with your fingers underneath for support and your thumbs on the top of the leg, just above the knee. Press inward two or three times, holding for three to five seconds each time.

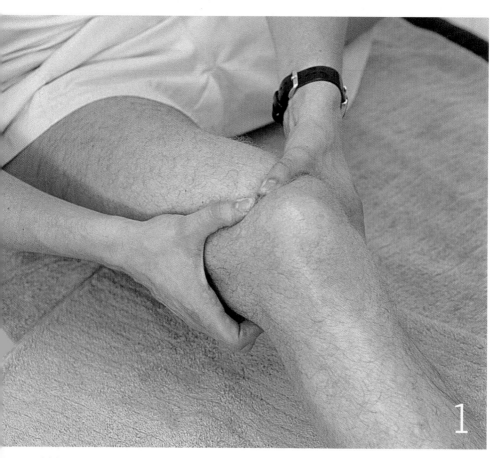

2

Holding the top of your knee with one hand for support, bend slightly and place the thumb of your other hand in the hollow above the ridge of the bone in the lower leg (femur) near the crease. As in step 1, press inward two or three times, holding the pressure for three to five seconds each time.

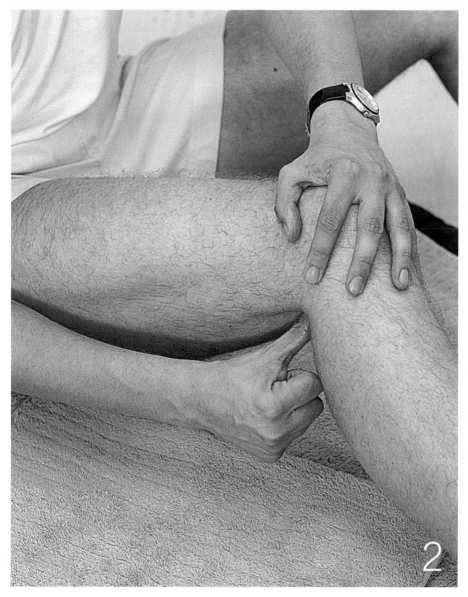

Aching Pecs

The broad, flat area at the front of the chest on either side of the breast bone houses the pectoral muscles, which connect the ribcage, the collar bone and the top of the bone in the upper arm (humerus) (see pages 15 and 16). Over-exercising the upper torso puts a strain on these large muscles and causes discomfort. This type of strain is a common occurrence for weight-lifters, body-builders and boxers.

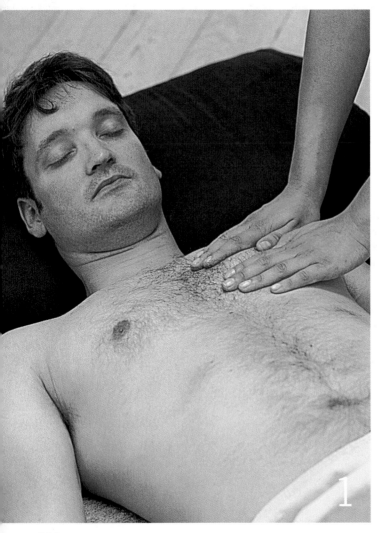

1

Working side-on to your partner, place the flat of both your hands on the central chest in line with the lower ribs and using effleurage (see page 24), glide your hands sideways up the chest, across the top of the shoulder to the outer edge and down the outer side of the upper torso, back to where you started.

Repeat several times.

2

Keeping one hand on the centre of his chest, place the hand nearest to your partner's head on the pectoral muscle furthest away from you and, using the whole hand but applying firm pressure from the heel, glide along the length of the muscle, stroking your fingers over the top of the arm. Return with less pressure.

Repeat several times.

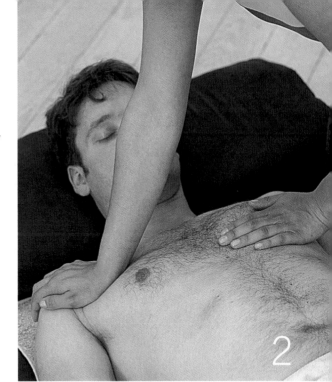

3

Moving to a position above your partner's head, lean forward and place your hands on the pectoral muscles, with your fingers pointing to the edge of his chest. With your arms straight, apply firm pressure and stretch each muscle with a slight push downward. Take care not to slide off, as this is a press-and-stretch move rather than a glide.

Repeat several times.

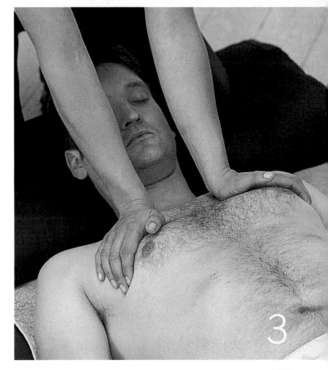

Tennis Elbow

As the name suggests, this complaint is associated with strenuous racket games such as tennis, and is caused by untreated tightness and over-straining of the wrist extensors or by nodules and lesions that make the muscles prone to injury. The initial sign of tennis elbow is an ache not at the elbow but in the mid-section of the forearm, which may wear off but returns each time the arm and wrist are used. In the worst case the wrist, rather than the elbow, needs to be immobilized for a period of time, but in most instances deep friction massage (see page 30) and manipulation of the joints will relieve the complaint.

1

Facing your partner, support her arm with your forearm and hold her elbow in your upturned, cupped hand.

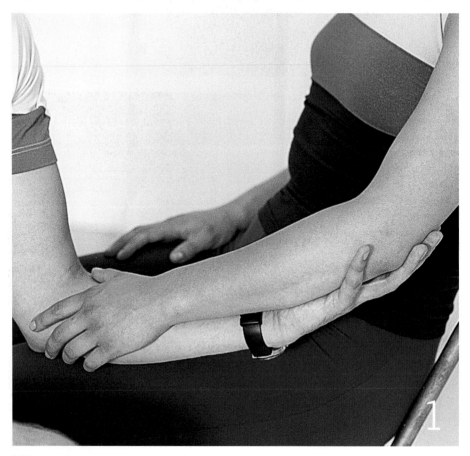

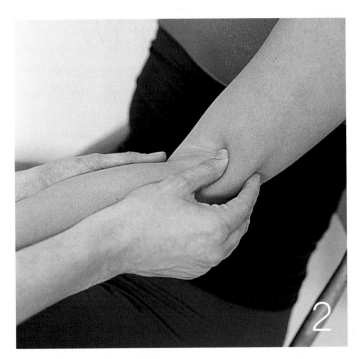

2

Place your thumb on the outside of the elbow with your fingers underneath to apply counter pressure and, working around the outside of the elbow, apply pressure with the pad of your thumb, rotating it at the same time.

3

With your hands in the same position as for step 2, use the tip of your thumb instead of the pad to apply pressure by moving it backward and forward across the elbow in short strokes. Continue for one to two minutes, or to your partner's tolerance level, as this stroke can cause some discomfort.

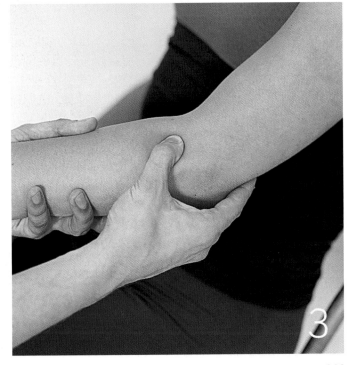

Golfer's Elbow

Like tennis elbow, the name describes a complaint suffered by people who play a particular sport, in this instance, golf. The causes are the same as for tennis elbow, but this time they relate to the upper arm. The symptoms are different from those of tennis elbow; the first sign of golfer's elbow is pain in the wrist joint when the elbow is extended and facing upward. Sufferers of golfer's elbow will find that during activity the upper arm will ache.

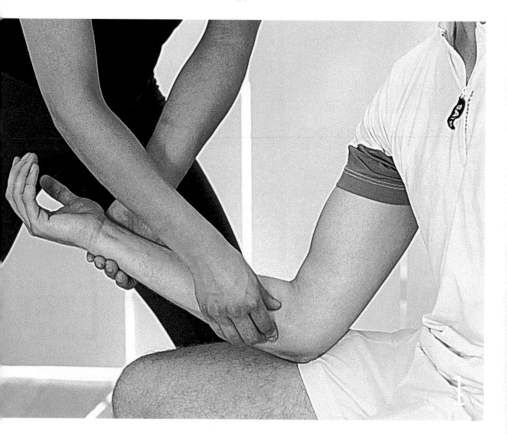

1

With your partner's arm facing upward, make sure the elbow is supported either on his thigh or on a stable surface and support his wrist with your hand.

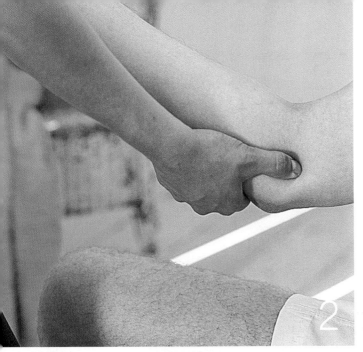

2

Place your thumb on the inside of the elbow and, working around the area, apply pressure with your thumb pad, rotating it at the same time.

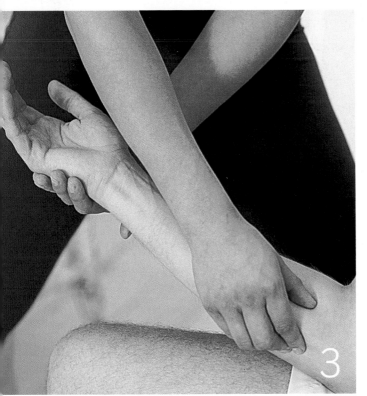

3

With your hands in the same position as for step 2, use your thumb tip instead of the pad to apply pressure by moving it backward and forward across the inside of the elbow in short strokes. As this area can be very tender, continue only to your partner's comfort level.

Frozen Shoulder

A pain in your shoulder as if you have slept awkwardly and then a sudden inability to lift your arm, accompanied by excruciating, deep burning pain are the symptoms of a frozen shoulder. This is caused by injury or repetitive exercise, and those over the age of 40 are more susceptible to the problem. Specialists stress the importance of early help, and one of the most effective treatments involves pressure and gradual stretching of the deep soft tissue and tendons.

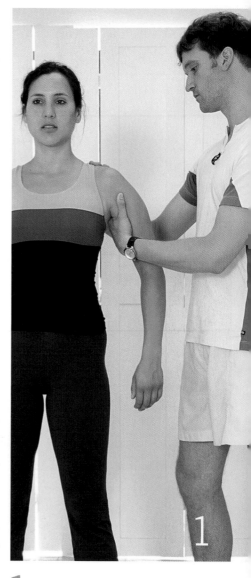

PROFESSIONAL HELP

If the symptoms have been left too long for home treatment, consult an osteopath who may be able to 'unfreeze' the shoulder over a series of treatments.

1

In a standing position, support your partner's upper arm with both hands and place one hand on the underside of the shoulder joint, lifting it very slightly. Move gently, as this action can feel very tender or even painful for your partner.

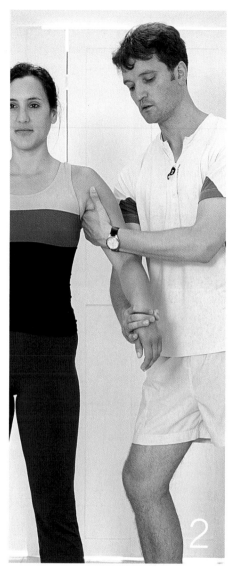

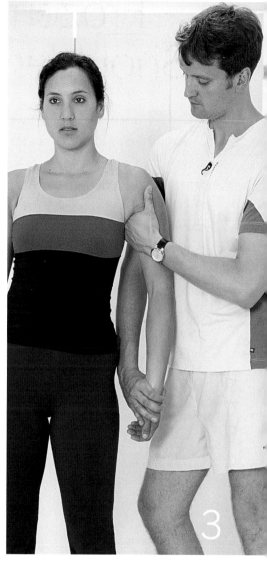

2

Keeping one hand under the arm, slide your other hand down to your partner's wrist for support and pull their straight arm forward and outward to a comfortable point of resistance. Warn your partner in advance to tell you as soon as this becomes too painful.

3

Keeping your hands in the same position as in step 2, pull outward with the hand under her shoulder, at the same time pulling down with the hand supporting her wrist. Hold the stretch for as long as your partner can tolerate, then release it.

Back Spasm

When a back is in spasm you cannot apply any deep strokes until the whole area has been warmed up and the muscles relaxed, so before a heavier stroking action a very light-pressured, criss-cross effleurage is used (see page 24). Once this has been completed you can continue with further treatment (see pages 52–5).

SELF-HELP BACK ROUTINE

The following easy routine helps the back as it relieves the pressure put on the intervertebral discs in standing and sitting positions. It allows the back muscles to relax and in doing so lengthens the spine and allows the flow of fluid to the centre of the discs, restoring their cushioning effect.

1 Wearing loose-fitting clothing, lie down on your back on the floor.

2 Make sure your head is well supported by a rolled-up towel or a pillow.

3 Bend your knees upward so that your feet are flat on the floor, and hip width apart.

4 Rest your hands on your hips, with your arms resting on the floor.

5 Let the lower part of your back make contact with the floor.

6 Close your eyes and hold the position for a count of 20.

7 Bring your knees up to your chest, hug them, and hold for a count of 20.

8 Return to the starting position and repeat twice more.

SAFETY FIRST

Remember: always work on either side of the spine, never directly over it.

1

Facing your partner side-on, place your hands on opposite sides of the lower back area on either side of the spine and apply the effleurage stroke (see page 24), gliding your hands across the back in opposite directions. Continue working up the back area to the top and then repeat back down to where you started. Keep your rhythm slow, taking four to five seconds to glide from one side of the torso to the other. The aim is to achieve relaxation rather than stimulation.

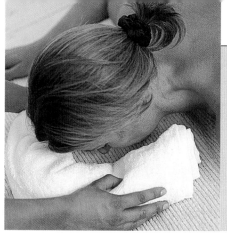

Tip
Folding a hand towel
into a horseshoe
shape creates a
comfortable support
for your partner's head
while you are working
on their back.

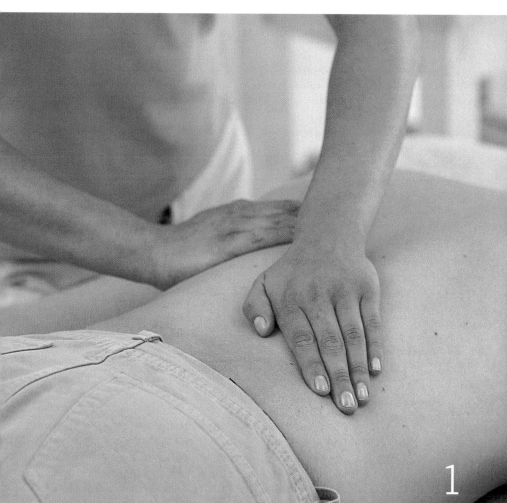

1

Index

Acknowledgments

All photography by **Octopus Publishing Group Ltd.**/Peter Pugh-Cook

Models: **Andrew Yhannakou** at Ugly Models, **Debbie B** at Model Plan, **Philomena Roullard**, **Nicole Uprichard**, **Robert Clarke**, **Nicky Ross**, **Lucy Moore**, baby **Oliver Dowling**

Executive Editor: **Jane McIntosh**
Editor: **Katy Denny**
Executive Art Editor: **Leigh Jones**
Production Controller: **Aileen O'Reilly**